Clinical
Naturopathy:
In Practice

Clinical Naturopathy:
In Practice

Jerome Sarris
Jon Wardle

ELSEVIER

ELSEVIER

Elsevier Australia. ACN 001 002 357
(a division of Reed International Books Australia Pty Ltd)
Tower 1, 475 Victoria Avenue, Chatswood, NSW 2067

Notice

Knowledge and best practice in this field are constantly changing. As new research and experience broaden our understanding, changes in research methods, professional practices, or medical treatment may become necessary.

Practitioners and researchers must always rely on their own experience and knowledge in evaluating and using any information, methods, compounds, or experiments described herein. In using such information or methods they should be mindful of their own safety and the safety of others, including parties for whom they have a professional responsibility.

With respect to any drug or pharmaceutical products identified, readers are advised to check the most current information provided (i) on procedures featured or (ii) by the manufacturer of each product to be administered, to verify the recommended dose or formula, the method and duration of administration, and contraindications. It is the responsibility of practitioners, relying on their own experience and knowledge of their patients, to make diagnoses, to determine dosages and the best treatment for each individual patient, and to take all appropriate safety precautions.

To the fullest extent of the law, neither the Publisher nor the authors, contributors, or editors, assume any liability for any injury and/or damage to persons or property as a matter of product liability, negligence or otherwise, or from any use or operation of any methods, products, instructions, or ideas contained in the material herein.

National Library of Australia Cataloguing-in-Publication Data

---

Sarris, Jerome, author.
Clinical naturopathy : in practice / Jerome Sarris, Jon Wardle.
9780729542128 (paperback)
Includes index.
Naturopathy.
    Clinical medicine.
Wardle, Jon, author.

Senior Content Strategist: Larissa Norrie
Content Development Specialist: Lauren Santos
Senior Project Manager: Anitha Rajarathnam
Edited by Matt Davies
Proofread by Tim Learner
Design by Lisa Petroff
Index by Innodata Indexing
Typeset by Toppan Best-set Premedia Limited
Printed in China

To my mother, Cynthia. Without her love and support my world would fall apart. To my sister, Ellena. Her familial enthusiasm, humour and creativity always inspire me.
– Jerome

For Kath and Molly.
– Jon

Contents

Editors

Jerome Sarris ND (ACNM), MHScHMed (UNE), AdvDipAcu (ACNM), DipNutri (ACNM), PhD (UQ)
Professor of Integrative Mental Health, NHMRC Clinical Research Fellow, NICM Deputy Director, Western Sydney University, New South Wales; Honorary Principal Research Fellow, Department of Psychiatry, The University of Melbourne, Victoria, Australia

Jon Wardle ND (ACNM), MPH (UQ), MHlthMedLaw (Melb), PhD (UQ)
Head, Regulatory, Policy and Legislative Stream, Australian Research Centre in Complementary and Integrative Medicine, Faculty of Health, University of Technology Sydney, New South Wales, Australia
Visiting Professor, School of Medicine, Boston University, Massachusetts, USA
Naturopathic Practitioner, Herbs on the Hill, Queensland, Australia

Preface

In our efforts to improve and modernise our seminal naturopathic text *Clinical Naturopathy: An Evidence-Based Guide to Practice*, we sought feedback from a variety of sources—including naturopathic students, naturopathic practitioners and lecturers within naturopathic programs in Australia and overseas. During these consultations the place of case studies repeatedly came up, in particular their importance in contextualising theoretical and 'evidence-based' information. Most of the people we contacted agreed on the importance of case studies, yet it was difficult to find agreement on how they would fit into the text.

Some suggested that the case studies were too descriptive and could be seen as summaries of the chapters, encouraging readers to follow the prescribed protocols rather than translate the chapter content into their own cases. Others highlighted how important it was to translate the chapter content into the context of real-life patients and to disseminate the wisdom that comes from practice, in addition to that which comes from theory and research. While some commended the ability of our case studies in the first edition to 'fit' nicely within the chapter topics, others felt conversely that this unnecessarily restricted the impact of the case studies by fitting them into topics, rather than treating them holistically as individual cases. While disagreement abounded, one thing became abundantly clear: case studies were far too important and complex to serve as supplementary material to place at the end of each chapter. The purpose of this text, therefore, is to recognise this importance and complexity of case studies and to 'unshackle' them from their supplementary role, developing them as important learning tools in their own right.

These cases are meant to illustrate the approaches of leading naturopathic practitioners in treating various conditions. They should not be seen as prescriptive—every case is unique after all—but they are meant to contextualise how research and theory have been applied in real-world settings by leading clinicians. Each of these cases is based on a real-world case, as treated by the author as a clinician. As such the text offers a great insight into the clinical decision-making processes of leading clinicians. By nature, this approach also highlights the breadth of treatment approaches in naturopathic practice (and clinical practice more broadly). These cases aren't 'right' or 'wrong' (although you can observe how the patient is expected to progress) but simply illustrative of the approaches used by these leading clinicians.

However, it should also be noted that due to various limitations (e.g. word count and generalisability to an extent), more complex cases have not been presented. More importantly the purpose was to provide case studies that are most generalisable to common conditions seen in clinical practice. It is acknowledged that patients present with individualised conditions and that each case is unique and often complex; however, it was felt that the lessons from practice could be maximised by highlighting those cases most likely to be encountered by naturopathic clinicians in their practice. We have also provided expected follow-up protocols in each of the cases to guide readers as to what to expect throughout the patient journey, whether that journey be long or short.

Readers will probably also notice that references have not been included in this book. Instead, a bibliography of relevant resources has been provided to assist those interested in the theory and research underlying these case studies. This should also be viewed in the context that the aim of this book is to disseminate the wisdom drawn from practical experience (the importance of which is further discussed in the introductory chapter) and, in this sense, serves as a complementary approach to the theoretical and research focus of *Clinical Naturopathy: An Evidence-Based Guide to Practice* (and other naturopathic and medical texts). We have also included clinical pearls and clinical comprehension questions—provided by authors—to help readers better understand practical concepts that drive the author's clinical decision making.

We believe that this text complements the existing literature, which often ignores clinical experience in favour of research and theory. By developing this text for use in addition to existing resources, we hope that readers can be exposed to a more rounded learning experience, ultimately delivering better clinical outcomes for patients.

Jerome Sarris
Jon Wardle
May 2017

Contributors

Susan Arentz ND, PhD, BHSc(Hons), AdvDipNat
Adjunct Research Fellow, NICM Western Sydney University, New South Wales, Australia
Lecturer, Endeavour College of Natural Medicine, New South Wales, Australia
Naturopath, Alana Healthcare for Women, New South Wales, Australia

Leslie Axelrod ND, LAc
Professor of Naturopathic Medicine, Department of Clinical Sciences, Southwest College of Naturopathic Medicine, Arizona, USA

Diana Bowman ND, PhD(c), MHSc, BHSc
Lecturer, Faculty of Health University Technology Sydney, New South Wales, Australia

Michelle Boyd ND, MHSc(HMed), BHSc(Nat), GradCert(HEd)
Medical Herbalist and Naturopath, Herbs on the Hill Clinic, Queensland, Australia

Joanne Bradbury ND, PhD(Nutritional Pharma), GradCertBiostats, BNat(Hons), BA(Psych)
Lecturer, Southern Cross University, Queensland, Australia

David Casteleijn ND, PhD(c), MHSc(HerbMed), BHSc(Nat)
Director and Clinician, Herbs on the Hill, Queensland, Australia
Lecturer, University of Technology Sydney, New South Wales, Australia

Kieran Cooley ND, BSc
Director, Research and Clinical Epidemiology, Canadian College of Naturopathic Medicine, Ontario, Canada

Phil Cottingham ND, BHSc, PGDip, GradDip
Principal, Wellpark College of Natural Therapies, Auckland, New Zealand

Sandy Davidson ND, PhD(c), DRM, MPH, AdvDipNat, DipNut
Program Leader, Nutritional Medicine, Endeavour College of Natural Health, New South Wales, Australia

Tessa Finney-Brown ND, MD, BHSc(Nat)

Jane Frawley ND, PhD
Lecturer, Public Health Faculty of Health, University of Technology Sydney, New South Wales, Australia

Stephanie Gadsden ND, GradCert(MH), BHSc(Nat)
Secretary (Board of Directors), International Network of Integrative Mental Health, New Jersey, USA
Director, Merge Health, Victoria, Australia

Neville Hartley ND, MPhil(Biomed), BHSc(CompMed)
Senior Lecturer, Health, Australasian College of Natural Therapies, Queensland, Australia

Jason Hawrelak ND, PhD, BNat(Hons), MASN, MNHAA, FACN
Senior Lecturer, Complementary and Alternative Medicines School of Medicine, University of Tasmania, Australia
Visiting Research Fellow, Australian Research Centre in Complementary and Integrative Medicine, University of Technology Sydney, New South Wales, Australia

Christina Kure ND, PhD, BAppSci
Research Fellow, Centre for Human Psychopharmacology, Swinburne University of Technology, Victoria, Australia

Matthew Leach ND, PhD, BN(Hons), DipClinNutr
Senior Research Fellow, Department of Rural Health, University of South Australia, Australia

Karen Martin ND, MDEd, BTeach(Adult)
Director and Naturopath, Well2 Pty Ltd, South Australia, Australia

Kathleen Murphy ND, BA, BHSc
Naturopath, MamaCare Health Services, New South Wales, Australia
Lecturer, Naturopathic Medicine, Endeavour College of Natural Health and Australasian College of Natural Therapies, New South Wales, Australia

Georgina Oliver ND, MSc, BHSc
Research Assistant, Department of Psychiatry, University of Melbourne, Victoria, Australia

Paul Orrock DO, ND, MAppSc, GradCertHEd
Senior Lecturer, Health and Human Sciences, Southern Cross University, New South Wales, Australia

Daniel Roytas ND, MHSc(Nat), BHSc
Clinician, Ultima Healthcare, Queensland, Australia

Ses Salmond ND, PhD
Herbalist, Naturopath, Homoeopath, Researcher, New South Wales, Australia

Janet Schloss PhD, PGCNut, AdvDipHS, BARM, DipNut, DipHM
Research Officer, Surveys and Statistics Office of Research, Endeavour College of Natural Health, Queensland, Australia

Justin Sinclair ND, DBM, DRM, FNHAA, MHerbMed, BHSc
Research Fellow, NICM Western Sydney University; Director & Principal Consultant, Traditional Medicine Consultancy; Lecturer, Naturopathic and Health Science Faculties, Australasian College of Natural Therapies, New South Wales; Lecturer, Naturopathic Faculty, Southern School of Natural Therapies, Victoria; Contract Academic, Naturopathic and Bioscience Departments, Endeavour College of Natural Health, New South Wales, Australia

Amie Steel ND, PhD, MPH, BHSc(Nat)
Postdoctoral Research Fellow, Australian Research Centre in Complementary and Integrative Medicine, University of Technology Sydney, New South Wales, Australia
Associate Director Research, Office of Research, Endeavour College of Natural Health, Queensland, Australia

Reviewers

Ayesha Amos
GradCertEvidCompMed, GradCertHEd, AdvDipAppSci(Nat)
Naturopathic Practitioner, North Coast Medical Centre, New South Wales; Lecturer, Australasian College of Natural Therapies, Queensland; Southern School of Natural Medicine, Victoria; Endeavour College of Natural Health, Queensland, Australia

Rachel Arthur
BNat(Hons) (1st class), BHSc
Private Practitioner, New South Wales, Australia

Lisa Costa Bir
GradDip(Nat), BAppSci(Nat), MATMS
Private Practitioner; Lecturer, Endeavour College of Natural Therapies, New South Wales, Australia

Emily Bradley
MNM, BHSc(Nat), ANTA
Naturopath, Clinic Supervisor, Stable Health Clinic; Lecturer, Southern School of Natural Medicine; Endeavour College of Natural Health, Victoria, Australia

Karen Bridgeman
ND, DBM, PhD, MSc(Hons), MEd(HEd), MAppSci, DipHom
Director, Starflower Pty Ltd, New South Wales, Australia

Robyn Carruthers
MHSc, BEd, AdvDipNat, AdvDipHerbMed, MNZAMH
Deputy Director, Clinical and Research, South Pacific College of Natural Medicine, Auckland, New Zealand

Thomas Harris
PhD, BSc(Hons), AdvDip(WestHerbMed)
Herbalist and Neuroscientist, Complex Health Management, Queensland, Australia

Nicole Quaife
BHSc(Nat)
Senior Lecturer, Nutrition and Nutritional Medicine, Laureate International Universities, Victoria, Australia

Michael Thomsen
ND, DBN, MSc
Medical Herbalist and Naturopath, Tasmania, Australia

Acknowledgments

Thanks are extended to the Elsevier team—Larissa Norrie, Lauren Santos, Anitha Rajarathnam and Neli Bryant. To the contributors, thanks for taking the bait to do this one!

Introduction
Evidence-based clinical naturopathic practice

Jon Wardle and Jerome Sarris

A resident, a junior attending physician, a senior attending physician and an emeritus professor were discussing evidence-based medicine. The resident passionately announced "EBM is a revolutionary development in medical practice, fundamental in solving patient problems". "A compelling exposition!" remarked the professor. "Hang on," the junior attending exclaimed, "EBM has merely provided a set of additional tools for traditional approaches to patient care". "A strong and convincing case!" the professor commented. "Their positions are diametrically opposed," exclaimed the senior attending, "they can't both be right." The professor looked thoughtfully at the puzzled doctor and replied, "You know what, you're right too!"[1]

The practice of naturopathy is developing from a traditional healing art into an evidence-based practice. As we stated in the preface to the first edition of *Clinical Naturopathy*, the increasing focus of evidence-based practice in the clinical application of naturopathy need not come at the expense of its intrinsic core principles. However, the constraints of a textbook project of that magnitude necessitated that the evidence base of the text focused on evidence from documentary sources—largely research papers but also traditional texts. We recognise that this approach had limitations. While the text reported in detail the clinical research evidence base for naturopathic practice, the insights drawn from clinical expertise garnered from years of practice were missing. With this case study book we hope to remedy this gap by providing examples drawn from the clinical experiences of leading practitioners to contextualise evidence within the practice setting.

These clinical insights are important to evidence-based practice. The 'father' of EBM, David Sackett, warned against the dogmatic application of EBM, noting that:

> ... good doctors use both individual clinical expertise and the best available external evidence, and neither alone is enough. Without clinical expertise, practice risks becoming tyrannised by evidence, for even excellent external evidence may be inapplicable to or inappropriate for an individual patient.

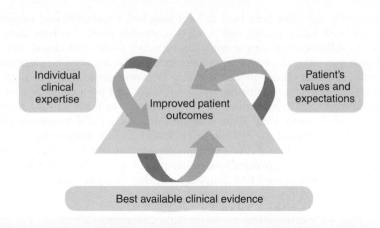

Figure 1: The evidence-based medicine 'triad'

Without current best evidence, practice risks becoming rapidly out of date, to the detriment of patients.[2]

Indeed, the EBM triad holds the best available clinical evidence, clinician expertise and respect for a patient's values and beliefs as three equally important aspects (see Fig. 1). At a clinical level, the defining features of *real* EBM are: making *ethical care* of the patient the top clinician priority; demanding *individualised evidence* in a form that both the clinician and the patient can understand; being characterised by *expert judgement* rather than mechanical rule-following; and *sharing clinical decision making* with patients via meaningful conversations.[3] The understanding of EBM as originally intended by David Sackett therefore guides the discussion of cases presented in this book.

Evidence-based medicine and naturopathic practice

EBM is an often poorly understood and maligned concept. Although only recently formalised, the concepts and principles of EBM have a long history, with the documented espousal of EBM principles (including the first documented description of a clinical trial) dating back at least to the writings of noted 10th century Islamic physician Avicenna—writings that went on to dominate Western medical training for more than 650 years.[4] In medicine, placebo controls were used in research as early as 1784, when a control was employed to explore (and later disprove) the medical effects of magnetism, a popular therapeutic system of the time,[5] but their political use predates their clinical use, being used by progressive Catholics in the 16th century to discredit right-wing exorcisms.[6] However, although many conflate EBM with the randomised controlled trials (RCTs) that often form a significant and influential part of EBM, there is much more to EBM than RCTs.

Naturopathy has often been held to have long had a turbulent and tumultuous relationship with EBM. Critics within the naturopathic profession have sometimes posited that EBM cannot coexist with naturopathy's philosophical and methodological underpinnings.[7] External critics have used similar arguments to suggest that naturopathy has little validity in contemporary evidence-based health practice.[8] Both arguments are incongruent with the reality of EBM, and proponents putting such arguments forward have bastardised the EBM concept to push forward their own vested interests. In truth, EBM aligns with the safe, effective and competent practice of naturopathy (or indeed any other health practice), and the notion that traditional knowledge or philosophies and scientific process cannot coexist is absurd. EBM is neither the bogeyman many detractors would paint it out to be, nor is it the rigid, inflexible system that many EBM 'proponents' (who, in reality, are not supporting *real* EBM at all) hold it to be.

What is evidence-based medicine?

The concept of EBM simply focuses on ensuring that clinical decisions about individual patients are made on the basis of the most up-to-date, solid, reliable, scientific evidence. Sackett's longstanding simple definition—still employed by most—is that 'EBM is the conscientious explicit and judicious use of the current best evidence in making decisions about the care of individual patients'.[2] *All* parts of this sentence are important. 'Current best evidence' is just that—not perfect evidence but simply the best up-to-date current evidence (not evidence that is out of date). And evidence extends not only to that found in academic journals but also that observed through clinical practice, uncovered through clinical expertise and even that found in long-standing traditions of safe and effective practice. This evidence must be applied in a 'conscientious' (i.e. being careful and thorough in all aspects of care), 'explicit' (i.e. clinicians must be open, clear, 'up-front' and transparent with patients in all aspects of their care) and 'judicious' (i.e. good judgement and common sense must be used in all clinical decision-making processes). And of course, it must be applied to 'individual' patients—including being respective of individual patient beliefs and preferences.

Evidence-based medicine in practice: key concepts

The key concepts of EBM in practice are not dissimilar to the concepts of good naturopathic practice. Indeed, many naturopathic clinicians will recognise many of the following concepts from their own practice. In practice, EBM requires that treatment be individualised, be clinically justified, follow proper procedures and focus on patient-centred outcomes.

Individualised treatment

One of the principal tenets of EBM is the encouragement of individualised treatment. Although EBM is often decried as encouraging 'cookbook' medicine, this arises from the discredited 'mechanical rule' interpretation of EBM; *real* EBM actually encourages an individualised approach.[3] The confusion possibly stems from EBM's use of protocols and clinical algorithms, which are often erroneously conflated as being 'cookbook' medicine. However, whereas 'cookbook' medicine provides a recipe of individual treatments that all patients within a subpopulation must be prescribed (for example, every patient with dysmenorrhoea must be prescribed *Vitex agnus-castus*), 'protocols' simply provide a standardised roadmap to treatment (for example, ensuring that: relevant differential diagnostic considerations are undertaken by performing relevant physical and diagnostic examinations; social and physical factors are taken into account; and all treatment groups have been considered). Similarly, EBM eschews the use of 'shotgun' approaches to treatment, whereby a prescription is provided that is so broad that it covers all possible bases, without differentiating what the patient actually *needs*. 'Shotgun' approaches to care not only expose patients to unnecessary clinical (i.e. potential interactions) and financial risk (which can result in resource constraints that make patients deter other necessary care),[9] they compromise quality continuity of care by making it difficult to ascertain which individual aspects of their treatment are actually working, making ongoing patient management problematic. They are also—to put it bluntly—an affront to the expertise of the clinician because they ignore the clinician's important role in tailoring an individualised prescription for the patient that is most likely to result in improved outcomes. They are also rarely as effective as individualised approaches to care.[10]

These 'shotgun' approaches are also worryingly present in many 'wellness' prescriptions—not *true* wellness prescriptions but those commercialised programs advising unnecessary use of a multitude of supplements without clinical justification—prescriptions that vary little between individual patients. In some cases, providing even seemingly benign unnecessary treatment can result in side effects that may mimic clinical symptoms. For example, one published case study reports of a British woman who had been unsuccessfully seeking treatment for unexplained peripheral neuropathy for 10 years as a result of a preventive 'shotgun' prescription approach to wellness that was not individually prescribed or well monitored, and contained high doses of pyridoxine.[11] Her symptoms immediately subsided on cessation of pyridoxine-containing supplements but after considerable resources had been expended on finding a cure for her symptoms.

Clinical justification for treatments

An obvious extension to individualised treatment is clinical justification of all treatments. While the importance of using individualised evidence has been discussed above, the clinical justification for treatment extends beyond clinical reasoning to ensuring that practice is also ethical. This principle is based on ensuring that treatments are derived in a 'conscientious, explicit and judicious' manner, not merely those based on personal preferences or interests. In naturopathic practice, practice dispensaries and the preponderance of availability of new diagnostic tests offer the following two case studies in how this may apply to clinical practice.

Proper procedures

Although 'mechanical rule following' is discouraged in *real* EBM, this does not mean that proper procedures and protocols should be discarded.[3] EBM even acknowledges that the procedures and processes may differ between differing levels of expertise.

While novice clinicians may work methodically and slowly through a long and standardised history and conduct an exhaustive physical examination and diagnostic tests, expert clinicians may make a rapid initial differential diagnosis through intuition, and then use a selective history, examination and set of tests to rule in or rule out particular possibilities.[3] The key similarity is that neither clinician relies on their knowledge or intuition alone and has strategies that confirm or deny their initial assumptions in a conscientious, explicit and judicious manner.

The importance of proper procedures and processes in EBM extends to the escalation of care. In clinical practice more invasive, expensive or risky procedures and treatments should never be considered first where less invasive, cheaper or safer procedures and treatments exist. In naturopathy, the therapeutic hierarchy[12] offers guidance to treatment and is itself an example of the sort of protocol encouraged by EBM. Similarly, no pathology test can replace a good case-taking technique or physical examination. Pathology tests should only ever be ordered once the information-gathering ability from these other sources has been exhausted.

Proper procedures must also be adhered to in relation to assessing evidence. While most people assume 'evidence' in EBM relates to the evidence supporting individual treatments, real EBM requires a risk–benefit assessment for all treatments. This necessitates not only a critical evaluation of the potential therapeutic benefits of the treatments proposed but also an assessment of the evidence for their *risks*. This risk–benefit assessment may change depending on individual patient circumstances. For example, a patient on a drug with a narrow therapeutic range (such as warfarin) may potentially be exposed to far more risk from interactive treatments than a patient on a drug with a broader therapeutic range. Warfarin, for example, may necessitate additional investigation or monitoring even in patients being recommended ordinarily benign therapies such as onion or green tea.[13] The spectrum of patient risk means that appropriate procedures concerning 'red flag' scenarios need to be incorporated into clinical practice.

Patient-centred outcomes

Real EBM is patient-centred. This, rather intuitively, simply means that outcomes from medical care are those that are important to patients. This is clearly apparent from 'patient values and expectations' forming an entire section of the EBM triad. Clinicians of all persuasions can be focused on what they see as clinically important outcomes, and real patient priorities may not always be apparent. Rheumatoid arthritis offers an insight into this disparity. While most clinical attention (and research focus) had been on reducing and managing the pain associated with this condition, patients are generally more concerned with the crippling fatigue associated with the condition.[14] Until qualitative work had uncovered this priority, most studies, and most treatment, had focused on what clinicians had thought was the obvious priority—pain.

Real EBM requires that the patient be heard and that the clinician treats *actual* patient priorities as identified by the patient, not just those the clinician *believes* are the most pertinent. The holistic and preventive focus of naturopathic medicine offers a further interesting example of patient priorities that can often be overlooked. Some clinicians may overlook immediate, acute or symptomatic treatment in favour of searching for the underlying cause that needs addressing. While identifying the underlying cause remains essential, it is unlikely to occur if the patient's immediate concerns are not also met. A patient presenting with an acute upper respiratory tract infection that is the result of reduced health (or 'vitality') caused by poor dietary and lifestyle behaviours is unlikely to comply with the dietary and lifestyle changes prescribed if their acute symptoms are not adequately treated. Pain (for example, dysmenorrhoea, migraine or rheumatoid arthritis) may have underlying triggers and exacerbating factors that can reduce the incidence, severity and impact on the patient long term but also require symptomatic relief during acute episodes.

What about traditional evidence?

Traditional knowledge, although often viewed as 'lower' on the evidence hierarchy, is not discounted by EBM entirely. Traditional evidence based on empirical observation over hundreds, sometimes thousands, of years can also be logically viewed as an extension of the 'clinician's experience' part of the EBM triad. However, there is growing international recognition of traditional medical knowledge as a source of evidence, as indicated in the World Health Organization's most recent *Traditional Medicine Strategy* document.[15] International efforts are underway to codify this traditional knowledge for greater recognition; for example, both traditional Chinese medicine and chiropractic diagnoses are being standardised for incorporation into the upcoming version of the *International Classification of Diseases*, which will give diagnoses from these medical traditions the same weight as 'Western' medical diagnoses.[16] In Australian courts traditional use and practice is already recognised as a form of admissible evidence, albeit at a lower level than scientific evidence.[17] Similarly, traditional evidence is also accepted by the Therapeutic Goods Administration, with protections against its fraudulent use (such as a requirement for documentation of multiple generations of use before allowing traditional evidence claims to be used so that traditions cannot be 'invented' for commercial or marketing purposes).[18]

Traditional knowledge is, in many ways, starting to be 'validated' by science. For example, while only now are the conditions in which a plant grows being recognised as a factor in their medicinal quality, this was long a part of herbal practice. In his 17th century treatise Nicholas Culpeper wrote of the conditions required for herbs to have optimal therapeutic qualities, noting in colewort's case that 'they rather delight to grow in shadowy than sunny places'.[19] Modern science is only now confirming why brahmi displays different therapeutic qualities depending on when it is harvested in relation to annual monsoons, as it has been known to do for centuries.[20] There are also important practical reasons for recognising tradition. The ban on kava (*Piper methysticum*) in many countries was triggered via hepatotoxicity occurring in rare cases. This primarily involved solvent-extracted German preparation using the incorrect plant parts and cultivars, rather than using traditional aqueous extractions of the rootstock of high-quality kava cultivars.[21] While the implementation within different countries varies—and varies considerably—groups such as the World Health Organization are recommending *more* recognition of traditional medical knowledge, not less.[15]

However, a reliance on traditional evidence alone is not enough in EBM. Just as an over-reliance on scientific evidence alone can result in practice being 'tyrannised by evidence', or an over-reliance on clinical expertise alone can result in practice becoming 'rapidly out of date',[2] relying solely or too much on traditional evidence can present its own problems. Real EBM requires the totality of all forms of evidence to be considered in every clinical encounter.

Limitations and problems in EBM

There are noted limitations in the application of EBM. Clinicians may denounce that, in many cases, the highest form of empirical study—the clinical trial—may not accurately reflect the true practice of therapies. There is a valid criticism that clinical trials too often measure the effects of therapies in a way it is never going to be used (many trials require the intervention be used exclusively or be applied to strictly controlled criteria rather than individual clinical judgement) in patients who are never going to be seen in a clinic (many trials exclude multimorbidity and patients with numerous health risk factors unrelated to the clinical condition being investigated) by physicians who will never actually practise (many trials do not use grassroots practitioners but researchers) in settings that don't actually exist (many trials take place in research centres rather than functioning clinics). Such criticisms are particularly pertinent to the naturopathic community, where the variation between a research setting and the 'real-world' practising environment may be particularly pronounced.[22]

However, such criticisms do not stem solely from the naturopathic community. While naturopathic medicine often attracts enough criticism and controversy to highlight issues first—serving somewhat as an 'EBM canary in the coal mine'—few therapies are found to be effective using narrow, dogmatic, reductionist approaches to EBM. For example, orthopaedic and sports medicine seems to have an even lower evidence base than the naturopathic therapies recently included in the Australian private health insurance natural therapies review.[23] Even primary care itself cannot survive this bastardised approach to EBM. Stange and colleagues draw attention to what they term the 'primary care paradox', noting that the complexities of primary care itself mean that its benefits can be obscured by dogmatic application of EBM— as studies that focus on narrow controlled interventions in patients that do not reflect the complexities, comorbidities and confounders observed in 'real-world' clinical practice.[10] As such, the benefits of primary care can differ depending on which evidence is being interpreted: trial evidence fairly consistently shows that primary care clinicians deliver poorer quality care than specialists; evidence from the Medical Outcomes Study, however, shows similar outcomes for specialists and generalists but at a lower cost for generalists (representing higher value); in studies of patients with chronic somatic and/or mental illness, shared care between specialists and generalists is optimal; ecological studies find that a greater supply of generalists and a lower supply of specialists is associated with greater quality of care on multiple disease-specific quality measures; ecological studies show that more primary care is associated with better population health with a lower cost and greater equity.[10]

However, in many cases, EBM is incorrectly perceived to align only with the first form of evidence (trials), potentially obscuring the value of primary care. However, the other forms of evidence listed are becoming increasingly important in clinical and policy decision making and have also been suggested to more accurately reflect the true principles and practices of naturopathic medicine.[24] It should be noted that such developments may not—yet—be fully embraced by the conventional medical community (the well-publicised methodological flaws with recent National Health and Medical Research Council (NHMRC) reviews of natural therapies is an obvious example). There have also, undoubtedly, been problems with misappropriation of EBM by various vested interests, from dogmatic fervent proponents pushing their own incorrect narrow interpretations of EBM, to drug companies influencing the research process (via development of new research tools, publication bias and invention of new 'conditions' requiring treatment) to better push their own products via the EBM model.[3] However, these problems aren't due to EBM but to its misappropriation and distortion by a vocal and influential minority.

The perceived conflict between naturopathy and EBM—is it really reflective?

The perceived conflict between naturopathic medicine and EBM appears to be a side effect of the political tensions between naturopathic and conventional medicine professions rather than a true conflict or inability for naturopathic medicine and EBM to align. The use of narrow and dogmatic (and false) interpretations of both EBM and science as blunt weapons against naturopathic medicine by ideological opponents (for example, by labelling them pseudoscientific and incompatible with conventional medical principles) have probably lent credence to this perceived conflict.[25] Some commentators within the naturopathic profession have been equally unhelpful, suggesting that any move to embrace EBM by Australian naturopathy, for example, is driven solely by political factors and that the idea of EBM aims at bypassing or minimising the philosophical and methodological foundations of naturopathy.[7] Some commentators have attempted to further dissociate EBM and complementary medicine as two distinct, separate and opposite entities—suggesting, for example, that the upsurge in the use of integrative therapies by conventional medical practitioners is linked to their defence of clinical autonomy in the face of pressures to practice an 'approved' version of EBM.[26]

However, the notion that the underlying principles, philosophies and practices of naturopathic medicine are too philosophically divergent to engage with EBM does not alter the reality of perceptions of grassroots naturopathic practitioners and students. Australian studies of naturopathic students[27] and practitioners[28] have suggested that practitioners critically engage with both traditional and scientific forms of evidence and with information that both supports and is critical of traditional naturopathic practices. This aligns with Boon's early Canadian work that suggested that naturopaths viewed treatment through a spectrum of scientific and holistic worldviews and were able and willing to be more holistic or more scientific depending on patient needs,[29] as well as international studies of the naturopathic profession's attitudes towards EBM.[30] It also aligns with data that suggests complementary professions in Australia—particularly Chinese medicine and naturopathy—are becoming more actively engaged and successful in health and medical research funding streams such as those of the NHMRC.[31]

Where is the evidence?

The largest problem facing naturopathic medicine with respect to evidence is not the negative evidence suggesting that naturopathic medicine does not work but the paucity of evidence at all. Even more pressing is the need for research around the practice of naturopathy, which can highlight the valuable role of the naturopathic clinician in delivering care rather than placing emphasis on the role of the therapy (e.g. herbal medicine, acupuncture, nutritional supplement) itself.[24] However, it is not the role of the scientific community to build naturopathy's evidence-base; it is the naturopathic community's obligation to build research capacity among its own clinicians and to build the evidence-base itself.[32,33] After all, no-one else can be expected to do it for us. Not only does this ensure that the naturopathic profession has a foundation upon which to base EBM but it also ensures that the evidence-base is truly reflective of naturopathic practice and respectful of naturopathic traditions.[34] This does not necessarily mean that clinicians should conduct their own projects, although this should be encouraged, but that a culture of involvement in ongoing projects should be supported, whether that be involvement in surveys, focus groups, trials or initiatives such as practice-based research networks (e.g. the Practitioner Research And Collaboration Initiative in Australia[35] or the Naturopathic Physicians Research Institute in the United States). If the naturopathic community does not establish its own evidence base, the vacuum will be filled by the misinformed assumptions of sceptical opponent groups, whose views will be lent more legitimacy than they deserve solely due to the fact that no opposing point of view has been established. This does not support the naturopathic professions and it does not support good patient care.

Conclusion

EBM, though often cast as a 'bogeyman', is simply an extension of good clinical practice. The fear of embracing EBM in naturopathic practice appears to be related to an oversimplified and narrow interpretation of EBM by both naturopathic proponents and opponents—an interpretation that bears little resemblance to the true principles of EBM. EBM is a far more complex concept than we tend to give it credit for: 'evidence' is not synonymous with 'RCT'—many other forms exist; scientific knowledge is not a substitute for traditional knowledge *and vice versa*; and traditional knowledge is not an 'inferior' or 'undeveloped' form of knowledge. Science and tradition can coexist in EBM. They have different aims and structures and make different contributions to knowledge. Professional opposition to EBM in the naturopathic profession has no philosophical or traditional base. In fact, it could be argued that only by embracing EBM can naturopathic clinicians truly embrace their own philosophies and traditions.

Acknowledgement

This chapter is a summary of an invited talk prepared for and initially presented by Dr Jon Wardle in 2013 at the New Zealand Association of Medical Herbalists Conference in Dunedin and later updated and presented at the International Congress of

Naturopathic Medicine (Paris), Woodford Folk Festival and various naturopathic colleges around Australasia, Africa, North America and Europe. A version of this talk has also been published in the *Australian Journal of Herbal Medicine*.

REFERENCES

1. Guyatt G, Haynes R, Jaeschke RZ, et al; for the Evidence-Based Medicine Working Group. Evidence-based medicine: principles for applying the users' guides to patient care. *JAMA*. 2000;284(10):1290-1296.

2. Sackett D, Rosenberg W, Gray J, et al. Evidence-based medicine: what it is and what it isn't. *BMJ*. 1996;312:71-72.

3. Greenhalgh P, Howick J, Maskey N. Evidence-based medicine: a movement in crisis? *BMJ*. 2014;348:g3725.

4. Daly W, Brater D. Medieval contributions to the search for truth in clinical medicine. *Perspect Biol Med*. 2000;43(4):530-534.

5. Kaptchuk T. Intentional ignorance: a history of blind assessment and placebo controls in medicine. *Bull Hist Med*. 1998;72(3):389-433.

6. Kaptchuk T, Kerr C, Zanger A. Placebo controls, exorcisms and the devil. *Lancet*. 2009;374(9697):1234-1235.

7. Jagtenberg T, Evans S, Grant A, et al. Evidence-based medicine and naturopathy. *J Altern Complement Med*. 2006;12(3):323-328.

8. Dwyer J. Good and bad medicine: science to promote the convergence of 'alternative' and orthodox medicine. *Med J Aust*. 2004;180:647-648.

9. Wardle J, Adams J. The indirect risks of traditional, complementary and integrative medicine. In: Adams J, Andrews G, Barnes J, et al, eds. *Traditional, Complementary and Integrative Medicine: An International Reader*. London: Palgrave Macmillan; 2012:212-219.

10. Stange K, Ferrer R. The paradox of primary care. *Ann Fam Med*. 2009;7(4):293-299.

11. Silva C, D'Cruz D. Pyridoxine toxicity courtesy of your local health food store. *Ann Rheum Dis*. 2006;65:1666-1667.

12. Zeff J, Snider P, Myers S. A hierarchy of healing: the therapeutic order. In: Pizzorno J, Murray M, eds. *Textbook of Natural Medicine*. St Louis: Churchill Livingstone; 2006:27-39.

13. Heck A, DeWitt B, Lukes A. Potential interactions between alternative therapies and warfarin. *Am J Health Syst Pharm*. 2000;57(13):1228-1230.

14. Hewlett S, Cockshott Z, Byron M, et al. Patients' perceptions of fatigue in rheumatoid arthritis: overwhelming, uncontrollable, ignored. *Arthritis Rheum*. 2005;53:697-702.

15. World Health Organization. *WHO Traditional Medicine Strategy 2014-2023*. Geneva: World Health Organization; 2013.

16. Morris W, Gomes S, Allen M. International classification of traditional medicine. *Glob Adv Health Med*. 2012;1(4):38-41.

17. Weir M, Wardle J, Marshall B, et al. Complementary medicine and consumer law. *Compet Consum Law J*. 2013;25:85-110.

18. Weir M, Wardle J, Marshall B, et al. Therapeutic goods law—consumer law and complementary medicine. *Bond Law Rev*. 2013;25:13-34.

19. Culpeper N. *The Complete Herbal*. London: W. Foulsham & Co; 1653.

20. Phrompittayarat W, Jetiyanon K, Wittaya-areekul S, et al. Influence of seasons, different plant parts, and plant growth stages on saponin quantity and distribution in *Bacopa monnieri*. *Warasan Songkhla Nakharin*. 2011;33(2):193.

21. Sarris J, Adams J, Wardle JL. Time for a reassessment of the use of kava in anxiety? *Complement Ther Med*. 2009;17(3):121-122.

22. Wardle J, Seely D. The challenges of traditional, complementary and integrative medicine research: a practitioner perspective. In: Adams J, Andrews G, Barnes J, et al, eds. *Traditional, Complementary and Integrative Medicine: An International Reader*. London: Palgrave Macmillan; 2012.

23. Lohmander L, Roos E. The evidence base for orthopaedics and sports medicine. *BMJ*. 2015;350:g7835.

24. Wardle J, Oberg E. The intersecting paradigms of naturopathic medicine and public health: opportunities for naturopathic medicine. *J Altern Complement Med.* 2011;17(11):1079-1084.

25. MacLennan A, Morrison R. Tertiary education institutions should not offer pseudoscientific medical courses: standing up for science. *MJA.* 2012;196(4):225-226.

26. Adams J. General practitioners, complementary therapies and evidence-based medicine: the defence of clinical autonomy. *Complement Ther Med.* 2000;8(4):248-252.

27. Wardle J, Sarris J. Student attitudes towards clinical teaching resources in complementary medicine: a focus group examination of Australian naturopathic medicine students. *Health Info Libr J.* 2013;31(2):123-132.

28. Steel A, Adams J. The application and value of information sources in clinical practice: an examination of the perspective of naturopaths. *Health Info Libr J.* 2011;28(2):110-118.

29. Boon H. Canadian naturopathic practitioners: holistic and scientific world views. *Soc Sci Med.* 1998;46:1213-1225.

30. Goldenberg J, Burlingham B, Guiltinan J, et al. Shifting attitudes towards research and evidence-based medicine within the naturopathic medical community: the power of people, money and acceptance. *Int J Naturopath Med.* 2013;6(1).

31. Wardle J, Adams J. Are the CAM professions engaging in high-level health and medical research? Trends in publicly funded complementary medicine research grants in Australia. *Complement Ther Med.* 2013;21(6):746-749.

32. Wardle J. Building integrative medicine's research capacity. *Adv Integr Med.* 2014;1(3):105-106.

33. Adams J, Sibbritt D, Broom A, et al. Research capacity building in traditional, complementary and integrative medicine: Grass-roots action towards a broader vision. In: Adams J, Andrews G, Barnes J, et al, eds. *Traditional, Complementary and Integrative Medicine: An International Reader.* Buckinghamshire: Palgrave Macmillan; 2012.

34. Adams J, Wardle J. Engaging practitioners in research. *J Complement Med.* 2009;8(5):5.

35. Steel A, Adams J, Sibbritt D. Developing a multi-modality complementary medicine practice-based research network: the PRACI project. *Adv Integr Med.* 2014;1(3):113-118.

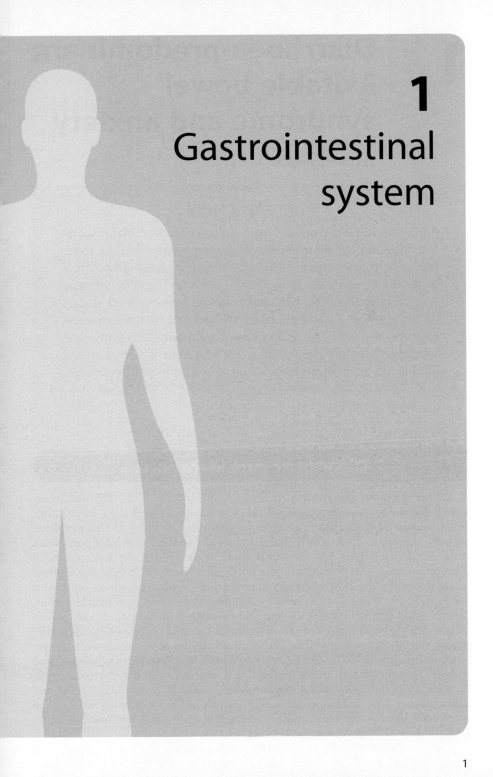

1
Gastrointestinal system

1 Diarrhoea-predominant irritable bowel syndrome and anxiety

Jason Hawrelak

PRESENTATION

A 34-year-old female presents with persistent **abdominal discomfort**, **bloating** and **diarrhoea**. Upon further questioning she states that on some days she does 3–4 bowel motions daily (Bristol Stool Scale type 6); other days only once. There is no blood in the stool, only occasional mucus. Gut symptoms are present on 3–4 days each week. She also complains of **anxiety** and believes **stressful episodes worsen her irritable bowel syndrome** (IBS) symptoms. Symptoms have persisted since a case of traveller's diarrhoea (and subsequent antibiotic treatment) she picked up in Bali 2 years ago.

Diagnostic considerations

While her symptom pattern does meet the Rome III criteria for IBS and, more specifically, diarrhoea-predominant irritable bowel syndrome (D-IBS), in cases like this a number of investigations need to be performed in order to rule out other potential diagnoses. Stool culture and parasitology (or faecal multiplex polymerase chain reaction (PCR)) needs to be performed to ascertain if any gastrointestinal pathogens remain from the original bout of traveller's diarrhoea in Bali. For accurate results this procedure may need to be done on three separate occasions, unless you use PCR, in which case a single sample will suffice. To rule out sugar malabsorption, breath testing (lactose and fructose) should be performed. Glucose breath testing should also be done to check for small intestinal bacterial overgrowth (SIBO). The patient should also be assessed for coeliac disease (note: to ensure an accurate test result, the patient needs to eat the equivalent of at least four slices of wheat bread daily for 6 weeks prior to coeliac testing). It is important to note that testing may find that a patient has multiples diagnoses such as SIBO, fructose intolerance and coeliac disease. Also be aware of alarm signs that require immediate referral such the presence of blood in the stool, unexplained weight loss, concurrent anaemia and a family history of bowel cancer.

MEDICAL CONDITIONS THAT MAY PRESENT AS D-IBS

- Coeliac disease
- Fructose intolerance
- Lactose intolerance
- SIBO
- Hyperthyroidism
- Chronic intestinal infections (bacterial or protozoan)
- Inflammatory bowel disease
- Colorectal cancer

Treatment protocol

- In this case, the results of the investigations did not alter the diagnosis, which remained D-IBS, and more specifically postinfectious D-IBS.

- One of the primary aims of treatment is to ensure gastrointestinal symptoms are reduced. This was achieved by using carminatives and antispasmodics (*Mentha x piperita, Lavandula* spp. and *Carum carvi*) and an antidiarrhoeal agent (*Myristica fragrans*). *Lactobacillus plantarum* 299v has also been found to decrease IBS symptoms—most notably abdominal pain and bloating—as well as decreasing stool frequency.

- To address the enhanced visceral perception, *Carum carvi* and *Mentha x piperita* were used in combination. The proprietary herbal preparation Iberogast has also been demonstrated to reduce visceral hypersensitivity.

- Turmeric was used to address the low-grade colonic inflammation that occurs in IBS and particularly in postinfectious IBS. *Lactobacillus plantarum* 299v administration has also been found to reduce inflammation in the colon.

- The underlying dysbiosis was addressed with galacto-oligosaccharides (GOS)—the prebiotic of choice in IBS. GOS reduce IBS symptomatology while simultaneously improving the gastrointestinal tract (GIT) microbiota. GOS supplementation has also been found to have an anxiolytic effect.

- *Schisandra chinensis* was used as an adaptogen to help modify the stress response. It has also been used in traditional Chinese medicine to treat diarrhoea and to 'calm and quiet the spirit'.

- The patient's comorbid anxiety was treated with relaxing nervines (*Lavandula angustifolia* and *Myristica fragrans*) and a nervous system trophorestorative (*Hypericum perforatum*). *Piper methysticum* is another herbal option that

3

can be very effective in helping to manage anxiety. Daily meditation was also recommended as a stress-minimisation strategy.

- *Hypericum perforatum* (St Johns wort) and *Myristica fragrans* (nutmeg) also have a long history of use in treating diarrhoea.

PRESCRIPTION
Herbal formula (100 mL)

Schisandra chinensis 1 : 2	25 mL
Carum carvi 1 : 2	20 mL
Mentha x piperita 1 : 2	15 mL
Hypericum perforatum 1 : 2	15 mL
Lavandula angustifolia 1 : 2	15 mL
Myristica fragrans 1 : 2	10 mL
Dose: 7.5 mL 2 × daily	

Nutritional prescription

Turmeric (curcumin phytosome): 1 capsule 2 × daily
Lactobacillus plantarum 299v 2 × 10^{10} CFU/day with a main meal
GOS: 3.5 g/day

Expected outcomes and follow-up protocols

IBS symptoms should substantially improve within 4 weeks (often earlier). Hence, follow-up should be scheduled in this time frame. The herb mix could be adjusted if the response was deemed inadequate at 4 weeks. If the patient was not responsive to treatment after 8 weeks, it would be worthwhile considering allergy testing (both IgG and IgE) to investigate the possible role of food allergies in their symptomatology. It should be noted, however, that a strict exclusion diet may be necessary to accurately ascertain which foods or food constituents are problematic in individual patients. A low-FODMAP diet could also be implemented, depending on the patient's initial response to treatment. It would also be worth considering the role of gluten in this case—even if coeliac testing was negative. Gluten sensitivity has been found to be a contributing factor to IBS symptoms in some patients. Unfortunately, there is no conclusive test for gluten sensitivity. Diagnosis is based on their response to a strict gluten-free diet and subsequent gluten challenge.

Both low-FODMAP and gluten-free diets have been found to negatively affect levels of beneficial bacteria in the GIT. A low-FODMAP diet should therefore be considered a short-term intervention until work on the underlying cause of the IBS symptoms and visceral hypersensitivity is completed. Healthy FODMAP-containing foods can then be slowly reintroduced into the diet. The patient's response to the gluten-free diet and gluten reintroduction will determine the length of time such a diet should be followed. If it is going to be followed long term, it is essential to provide dietary counselling to ensure an adequate amount and variety of dietary fibres and microbiota-nourishing foods are consumed daily to maintain a diverse and healthy GIT microbiota.

While symptoms can improve relatively quickly once treatment has begun, the underlying visceral hypersensitivity and colonic inflammation will take a number of months of ongoing treatment to heal. Once healed, most patients find they can eat a broad range of foods again without getting symptoms. These foods include fructose- and sorbitol-rich fruits, onions and legumes. Nervines and adaptogens provide restoration over the long term, so their use should be continued until both the practitioner and the patient are confident that they are no longer needed.

Clinical pearls

- IBS is still a diagnosis of exclusion. Ensure you've ruled out other possible diagnoses before assuming a patient has IBS.

- Always ask patients if there are any food triggers that they've observed for their gastrointestinal symptoms. These observations can give insight into what food constituents (if any) are causing problems for them.

- SIBO should be suspected in patients where bloating and distension are key symptoms—especially if these occur within 30 minutes of meals.

- Try to ascertain if there was an initiating event for their symptoms or what was happening in their lives around the time symptoms started. This can provide further insight as to the cause of gastrointestinal symptoms in that patient.

Expert | CONSULT

Clinical Comprehension Questions & Answers are hosted on **https://expertconsult.inkling.com/store/book/ sarris-clinical-naturopathy-case-files-1**

BIBLIOGRAPHY

Hawrelak JA. Irritable bowel syndrome. In: Wardle J, Sarris J, eds. *Clinical Naturopathy: An Evidence-Based Guide to Practice.* 2nd ed. Elsevier; 2014:73-100.

Lomer MCE. Review article: the aetiology, diagnosis, mechanisms and clinical evidence for food intolerance. *Aliment Pharmacol Ther.* 2015;41:262-275.

Shahbazkhani B, Sadeghi A, Malekzadeh R, et al. Non-celiac gluten sensitivity has narrowed the spectrum of irritable bowel syndrome: A double-blind randomized, placebo-controlled trial. *Nutrients.* 2015;7(6):4542-4554.

Silk DB, Davis A, Vulevic J, et al. Clinical trial: the effects of a trans-galactooligosaccharide prebiotic on faecal microbiota and symptoms in irritable bowel syndrome. *Aliment Pharmacol Ther.* 2009;29:508-518.

2 Gastro-oesophageal reflux disease and functional constipation

Jason Hawrelak

PRESENTATION

A 46-year-old female presents with a 3-month history of **retrosternal burning and regurgitation**. This occurs most days, and episodes can last up to 8 hours. The **burning pain improves upon antacid administration**, but she does not want to take these long term. She also has a long history of **constipation**. In fact, she can go 9 days between motions at times. When they do occur they are very pebbly and hard to pass (Bristol Stool Scale type 1). During the episodes of constipation she also suffers from **abdominal bloating and cramping**. Upon analysing her diet, it was found to fit the standard Australian diet—being low in fruits, vegetables and whole grains and high in caffeine and alcohol.

CLINICAL MANIFESTATIONS OF GORD

Classic symptoms
- Retrosternal burning sensation
- Regurgitation

Less common symptoms
- Dysphagia
- Cough
- Wheeze
- Laryngitis
- Dental erosions
- Noncardiac chest pain

It is also important to note that the severity of GORD symptoms is not a reliable indicator of the severity of the damage to the oesophagus.

Diagnostic considerations

The presentation of gastro-oesophageal reflux disease (GORD) is often classic and in these cases can be clinically confirmed by a positive acute response to antacids or gastrointestinal demulcents. In patients who present uncharacteristically or with a mixture of gastrointestinal symptoms, other diagnoses must be considered and ruled out. Referral for specialist investigative techniques (e.g. an endoscopy) may be required in these cases to accurately diagnose the clinical presentation.

Treatment protocol

- Providing acute symptomatic relief is paramount in managing GORD. A gastrointestinal demulcent (powdered marshmallow root, *Althaea officinalis* radix) was prescribed to acutely relieve the reflux symptoms and to help protect and heal the oesophageal mucosa. Powdered *Ulmus rubra* bark could also be used. Demulcent herbs provided as powders effectively coat the oesophagus to prevent contact between the inflamed mucosa and gastric acid; teas and tinctures will not provide this coating effect to the same degree.

- *Filipendula ulmaria* (meadowsweet) tea was prescribed to help decrease any oesophageal inflammation and to heal the mucosa. Teas are preferable to tinctures in GORD cases, as alcohol can have an exacerbating effect on GORD symptoms.

- A number of exacerbating lifestyle and dietary factors were discovered upon history taking. She consumed caffeine-containing beverages with most meals, ate lots of fatty foods, consumed wine most evenings after dinner, and ate snacks just before going to bed most evenings. To address these GORD risk factors, she was advised not to have any beverages with her meals and to drink fluids only between meals ($\geq$ 1 hour before or $\geq$ 2 hours after) to eliminate all caffeinated and alcoholic beverages, and to avoid other foods known to decrease lower oesophageal sphincter (LOS) pressure (peppermint lollies and chocolate). She was also advised to eat her evening meals earlier (prior to 7 pm), eat smaller meals in general and to not snack after 7 pm. Importantly, her water intake was assessed as adequate.

- To promote her antioxidant defences and prevent the development of Barrett's oesophagus, she was advised to consume more fruit daily (3–5 pieces), vegetables (five serves daily) and colourful whole grains (e.g. black and red rice). Foods rich in carotenoids and polyphenols were specifically recommended, as were kiwifruit, prunes and blackberries, as these three are all rich in antioxidants and may help promote bowel regularity.

- To increase gut transit time, the probiotic strain *Bifidobacterium animalis* DN-173 010 was used, which has been shown to significantly speed gastrointestinal tract (GIT) transit, as well as decreasing symptoms such as bloating and abdominal discomfort.
- Freshly ground flaxseeds were recommended for their bulking laxative effects. These were added to yoghurt.
- She was also advised to go for a daily walk in the mornings in an effort to get her bowels moving more regularly.

PRESCRIPTION
Herbal formula

Filipendula ulmaria: 2–4 cups daily between meals using 1 heaped tbsp per cup
GI demulcent powder: *Althaea officinalis* radix—1 heaped tsp mixed into a little water after breakfast, lunch and dinner, and as needed for acute relief of reflux symptoms

Nutritional prescription

Bifidobacterium animalis DN-173 010 1.25×10^9 CFU/day in a yoghurt medium
Ground flaxseeds: 2 tbsp daily mixed in with the yoghurt

Expected outcomes and follow-up protocols

If the patient successfully implements the dietary recommendations, the GORD symptoms should progressively abate over the course of the following weeks. Using a demulcent powder will usually relieve reflux symptoms within minutes of ingestion. The signposts of recovery will be a lessening of digestive discomfort and a reduction of regurgitation and other symptoms such as cough. After cessation of symptoms, the dietary recommendations, the *Filipendula ulmaria* tea and the gastrointestinal-demulcent powder should be continued to ensure healing of the oesophageal mucosa. After about 1 month without symptoms the demulcent powder can be used only as required, although the dietary modifications should continue. The practitioner should be aware that patients may fall back into poor dietary habits from time to time (such as drinking excess alcohol or eating known dietary triggers), so understanding and patience is required with the therapeutic relationship. In those patients who are unresponsive to initial therapeutic approaches, other diagnoses should be revisited (e.g. eosinophilic oesophagitis), the role of other potential contributing factors should be examined (e.g. gluten) and other therapeutic options should be considered (e.g. melatonin, 5-HTP or chiropractic/osteopathic manipulation for a hiatal hernia). It is important to note that, left untreated or poorly managed, long-term GORD can result in Barrett's oesophagus and a resultant increased risk of oesophageal cancer. Patients with definitively diagnosed or suspected GORD who do not respond to treatment should be referred on to a medical practitioner for follow-up assessment.

Constipation typically responds well to the combination of increased exercise, increased fruit, vegetable and whole grain intake, and ground flaxseeds. The addition of a probiotic strain that speeds gut transit time will further enhance the efficacy of this approach. Bowel movement frequency typically improves substantially within 2 weeks of beginning treatment. The additional use of stimulating laxative herbs is sometimes, although rarely, needed. In many constipation cases the symptoms of bloating and abdominal discomfort are secondary to the constipation. Once the bowels begin moving regularly, these symptoms typically cease or, at the least, improve considerably.

It is worth noting, however, that some patients with long-term constipation do not respond to the typical dietary approach detailed above. In many cases these individuals are found (through breath testing) to be high methane producers. Methane gas, in larger amounts, slows gastrointestinal transit time in some people. These patients require a different approach focused on suppressing the overgrowth of methane-producing bacteria within the GIT using specific prebiotic fibres and targeted antimicrobial agents.

Clinical pearls

- GORD is typically diagnosed based on the presence of classic symptoms (heartburn or regurgitation) but can also present with extraoesophageal manifestations such as a chronic cough or recurrent laryngitis as the main presenting complaint.

- GORD symptoms typically respond quickly to powdered gastrointestinal demulcents.

- Relief of retrosternal burning pain within minutes of administering demulcents can help to confirm a GORD diagnosis.

Expert|CONSULT

Clinical Comprehension Questions & Answers are hosted on
https://expertconsult.inkling.com/store/book/
sarris-clinical-naturopathy-case-files-1

BIBLIOGRAPHY

Dimidi E, Christodoulides S, Fragkos KC, et al. The effect of probiotics on functional constipation in adults: a systematic review and meta-analysis of randomized controlled trials. *Am J Clin Nutr.* 2014;100(4):1075-1084.

Hawrelak JA. Gastro-oesophageal reflux disease. In: Wardle J, Sarris J, eds. *Clinical Naturopathy: An Evidence-Based Guide to Practice.* 2nd ed. Elsevier; 2014:101-117.

Hawrelak JA. Irritable bowel syndrome. In: Wardle J, Sarris J, eds. *Clinical Naturopathy: An Evidence-Based Guide to Practice.* 2nd ed. Elsevier; 2014:73-100.

Kubo A, Corley DA, Jensen CD, et al. Dietary factors and the risks of oesophageal adenocarcinoma and Barrett's oesophagus. *Nutr Res Rev.* 2010;23(2):230-246.

3 Food intolerance

Jane Frawley

PRESENTATION

A 26-year-old woman presents with **diarrhoea, abdominal pain** and **flatulence** after eating different fruits and some dairy products. She explains that her stool is always very loose, with occasional bouts of **watery diarrhoea**. The **pain** (described as cramping) is under the umbilicus and worse in the lower left quadrant. She describes her flatulence as excessive and foul smelling and has a history of **gut sensitivity**. She has had various past investigations such as a colonoscopy (bowel mucosa normal), stool test (negative) and gliadin antibodies (negative). Past medications have included antibiotics occasionally for **sinusitis**.

Diagnostic considerations

The presence of recurrent diarrhoea, abdominal pain and excessive flatulence indicates disordered digestion. Long-term diarrhoea has many health consequences, such as dehydration and fatigue, and it is fundamental to determine the cause of the diarrhoea and treat it accordingly.

The presentation of diarrhoea in this case is chronic and therefore infectious bacterial and viral aetiology can most likely be excluded. The patient has also recently had a stool test that was negative for parasites. While this aetiology will be excluded for now, stool parasitology tests sometimes return false negative results and, if symptoms remain, follow-up testing may be required. The patient has also had a colonoscopy and gliadin antibodies were not found in a blood test, so coeliac disease can be discounted.

The patient's symptoms appear to be induced by eating, and because the flatulence is severe, it is wise to investigate intolerance to short-chain carbohydrates such as lactose and fructose. Maldigested lactose and fructose travel further down the digestive tract to the large bowel where they are used as a food source by colonic flora causing a build-up of gas and leading to pain and osmotic diarrhoea. Symptoms suggestive of fructose or lactose malabsorption include abdominal bloating, abdominal distension, abdominal pain, excessive flatulence, the onset of symptoms after eating, loose stool and diarrhoea. The presence of lactose and fructose malabsorption can be determined by a breath test, which is the initial consideration for this case. Treatment also involves herbal medicines for the symptomatic relief of flatulence, distension and pain associated with the condition, along with supplements to enhance the healing of the gut wall after problematic foods have been removed from the diet. The patient also indicates that she has had occasional antibiotics for sinusitis. Depending on the type, duration and frequency, these may have reduced certain populations of beneficial anaerobic bacteria in the gut.

MEDICAL CONDITIONS THAT MAY BE ASSOCIATED WITH OR AGGRAVATE DIARRHOEA

- Hyperthyroidism
- Coeliac disease
- Crohn's disease
- Ulcerative colitis
- Lactose intolerance
- Diverticulitis
- Bowel cancer
- Parasite infestation
- Gastroenteritis
- Food poisoning
- Irritable bowel syndrome
- Laxative abuse
- Alcoholism
- Excessive caffeine intake

Treatment protocol

- The patient is given a herbal formula containing *Mentha x piperita*, *Matricaria recutita*, *Melissa officinalis* and *Foeniculum vulgare* (for their carminative properties) and advised to take 5 mL three times a day to relieve the abdominal symptoms of distension, bloating and flatulence.

- The patient may have intestinal hyperpermeability due to the amount of time she has suffered from these gastrointestinal problems. She is prescribed glutamine (1000 mg/day), zinc (20 mg/day) and *Ulmus rubra* (1 tsp powered bark 3 × daily) to help with this.

- Test results revealed fructose and lactose malabsorption, therefore dietary advice is crucial and a low-fructose and low-lactose diet was prescribed, specifically, eliminating foods that contain fructose in higher or equal amounts than glucose such as apple, coconut (also coconut milk and cream), grape, guava, honeydew melon, mango, nashi fruit, paw paw/

papaya, pear, quince, star fruit, tomato and watermelon. She should also avoid fruit juice, fruit juice concentrate, dried fruit and tinned fruit. Vegetables such as Lebanese cucumber and sweet potatoes need to be avoided, along with condiments and miscellaneous items such as tomato sauce, tomato paste, chutney, relish, plum sauce, sweet and sour sauce, BBQ sauce, high-fructose corn syrup, fructose, honey and fortified wines. Stone fruits such as peaches, plums and apricots contain sorbitol, which can have similar effects on the gastrointestinal system as free fructose, so effects should be observed.

- Avoidance of fructan (chains of fructose units)-containing foods such as artichokes, asparagus, garlic, green beans, leek, onion, spring onion, shallots and wheat (many breakfast cereals, bread, biscuits, crackers, cakes, pies, pastas, pizzas and some noodles contain wheat) is also advised. Inulin and fructo-oligosaccharides should also be avoided. These commonly occur in health food products and prebiotic formulas. Foods such as rye, barley, banana and lettuce all contain fructans, but many people appear to tolerate moderate levels of these foods. Avoid initially, then reintroduce and observe.

- Avoidance of foods that contain more than 7 g of lactose per serve, which include cow's milk, sheep's milk and goat's milk (more than 1/3 of a cup on average), yoghurt (more than 100 g), ice-cream, cream cheese (more than 100 g) and cream-cheese-based dips is also recommended. Exercise caution with low-fat milk and cheddar cheese because some contain high amounts of lactose.

- Advising the patient to keep a food/symptom diary may also be a useful way to determine any other problematic foods.

PRESCRIPTION
Herbal formula (100 mL)

Mentha x piperita 1:2	20 mL
Matricaria recutita 1:2	30 mL
Melissa officinalis 1:2	25 mL
Foeniculum vulgare 1:2	25 mL
Dose: 5 mL 3 × daily	

Nutritional supplementation

Glutamine 1000 mg/day
Zinc 20 mg/day
Ulmus rubra 1 tsp 3 × daily

Lifestyle prescription

Dietary changes to avoid a high-fructose and -lactose diet

Expected outcomes and follow-up protocols

It is expected that abdominal symptoms such as distension and flatulence would be alleviated within 2 or 3 weeks of adhering to a fructose- and lactose-free diet. The herbal mix should also help to reduce these symptoms while the causes are rectified. If worrying symptoms such as diarrhoea are still present the patient needs to be referred for further testing.

In the case of lactose intolerance, it is important to determine if the intolerance is a primary or secondary intolerance. If the patient does not produce lactate the condition is a primary lactate deficiency (or lactose intolerance); however, for many people it is a secondary condition that is present as a result of other factors such as gastrointestinal inflammation. It is also important to keep small amounts of lactose in the diet (if not allergic to dairy foods) so that lactate continues to be produced; lifelong avoidance of dairy foods is not recommended. Additionally, while autosomal fructose intolerance exists it is a rare condition that is usually diagnosed in early childhood due to failure to thrive, hypoglycaemia and jaundice. Fructose malabsorption in an adult is usually a secondary condition and, as such, the goal is to reintroduce fructose-containing foods once they can be tolerated. Once the high-lactose and high-fructose foods are removed from the diet the small intestine is able to heal, and these foods can be reintroduced to the diet slowly in due course. Probiotics may also be of benefit if required, especially as many prebiotic foods may contribute to symptoms initially.

Clinical pearls

- It is always important to determine the source of diarrhoea because it is debilitating and may indicate a serious disorder such as ulcerative colitis, Crohn's disease, hyperthyroidism or bowel cancer.

- The addition of any new medication—natural or otherwise—should be investigated to ensure it is not contributing to the patient's symptoms.

- It is important to correctly diagnose food intolerances or allergies. Restrictive diets that are unnecessary are problematic for a variety of social, physical and psychological reasons.

- The ultimate goal is to reintroduce all lactose- and fructose-containing foods because they are important for a healthy, balanced diet.

Expert|CONSULT

Clinical Comprehension Questions & Answers are hosted on
**https://expertconsult.inkling.com/store/book/
sarris-clinical-naturopathy-case-files-1**

BIBLIOGRAPHY

Fedewa A, Rao SS. Dietary fructose intolerance, fructan intolerance and FODMAPs. *Curr Gastroenterol Rep.* 2014;16(1):1-8.

Frawley J. Food allergy/intolerance. In: Sarris J, Wardle J, eds. *Clinical Naturopathy: An Evidence-Based Guide to Practice.* 2nd ed. Sydney: Elsevier; 2014.

Gibson PR, Muir JG, Newnham ED. Other dietary confounders: FODMAPS et al. *Dig Dis.* 2015;33(2):269-276.

Mattar R, de Campos Mazo DF, Carrilho FJ. Lactose intolerance: diagnosis, genetic, and clinical factors. *Clin Exp Gastroenterol.* 2012;5:113.

4

Gastritis

Sandy Davidson

PRESENTATION

A 26-year-old female presents with **gastritis**, recently diagnosed subsequent to endoscopy and biopsy investigation. Results from the biopsy and blood sample were **negative for *Helicobacter pylori***. Symptoms have been present for approximately 6 weeks before diagnosis and include **gnawing diffuse gastric pain** described as severe and dyspepsia. She says it feels like a **knot in her stomach**. She has two to three episodes of severe pain daily while at work. Symptoms are worse for walking, hunger, red wine and spicy food and relieved by bland food, especially bread. She has gained 15 kg over the past 5 years; however, over the past 6 weeks she has lost 5 kg. She has a **high stress load** that exacerbates symptoms. She also experiences weekly **migraine headaches** that start as tension headaches and are **bilateral and throbbing** in nature. Recent blood pathology also revealed **prediabetes** and **elevated white blood cells**. All other routine blood pathology results were normal. Her GP recommended a low glycaemic index diet, which she is having difficulty implementing at the moment.

Diagnostic considerations

Primary treatment for the above case should involve resolving the gastritis and alleviating abdominal discomfort. The migraines have been investigated medically, and organic causes have been excluded. It is likely that her migraines are multifactorial in origin. Probable contributing factors are insulin resistance, food sensitivities and liver dysfunction triggered by her previous exhausting work environment. Although ibuprofen, alcohol and spicy foods are the most likely contributors to acute gastritis in this patient, there are a range of predisposing factors in the case that warrant screening to exclude cholelithiasis or gallbladder involvement. This could potentially be the underlying cause of gastritis in the absence of *Helicobacter pylori*. Although

15

her prediabetes state is of concern and requires attention, resolution of gastritis is the highest priority. To foster dietary adherence to a low glycaemic index and low glycaemic load diet, gastric symptoms must be resolved. Therefore once the gastritis symptoms have ceased focus would shift to weight management and blood glucose control.

MEDICAL CONDITIONS THAT MAY BE ASSOCIATED WITH OR AGGRAVATE GASTRITIS

- Nonsteroidal anti-inflammatory drugs including ibuprofen
- Alcohol
- Spicy foods such as chili
- *Helicobacter pylori* infection
- Gastric ulcer
- Coeliac disease
- Viral gastritis
- Parasitic infections
- Cholecystitis
- Cholelithiasis
- Viral gastroenteritis
- Crohn's disease

Treatment protocol

- The primary approach for herbal treatment is to reduce inflammation and heal the gastric mucosa. This is achieved through anti-inflammatory, vulnerary, carminative and demulcent herbs. These include the following:
  - *Matricaria recutita* optimises healing via down-regulation of TNF-α and reduction of apoptosis in the epithelial cells, which support its anti-inflammatory and vulnerary properties. It is an antispasmodic, carminative and nervous system sedative that may help relieve gastrointestinal discomfort and relax the central nervous system.
  - *Filipendula ulmaria* is a herbal antacid and analgesic with anti-inflammatory effects that reduces complement activity and T-cell activity.
  - *Glycyrrhiza glabra* is important not only due to its mucoprotective, anti-inflammatory and anti-ulcer effects but also for supporting a healthy stress response.
  - *Curcuma longa* in an anti-inflammatory and antioxidant.

- *Calendula officinalis* is recommended for treating inflammation of mucosa surfaces and to aid healing.
- *Tanacetum parthenium* inhibits phospholipase and prevents the release of 5-HT from platelets and polymorphonuclear leukocytes—a key target for neurovascular headaches and migraines. The herb is also highly indicated for inflammatory states.
- *Ulmus rubra* (inner bark) is prescribed for its mucilaginous and nutritive properties, providing a soothing and protective coat on gastric mucosal surfaces and enhancing nutrition. It has also demonstrated antioxidant activity in vitro in managing inflammatory bowel disease.
- Alpha lipoic acid facilitates the translocation of GLUT4 transporter to the cell membrane, enhancing glucose update and, with its potent antioxidant activity, will also support healing of gastric mucosa. Alpha lipoic acid has also been found to reduce migraine frequency, particularly if it is associated with dysglycaemia.
- Some studies have indicated that magnesium reduces migraine frequency and therefore is useful in migraine prophylaxis. The reduction in migraine frequency is thought to be attributed to a reduction of neuroexcitability and correcting mitochondrial dysfunction. Research has found that magnesium levels in migraine sufferers are lower than the normal range. Correction of mitochondrial dysfunction may also enhance insulin sensitivity.
- Dietary recommendations are important and include eliminating all aggravating substances for 6 weeks. These include ibuprofen, alcohol, coffee, chilli and garlic. Soft and easily digestible foods are recommended—examples include bone broths, fish soup, cabbage soup, porridge and casseroles. These foods are soothing and healing to gastric mucosa. Foods high in saturated fats, such as ghee, fried foods red meat and foods cooked in a lot of oil, should be reduced or eliminated.
- Taking an Epsom salt bath three times per week is recommended. This will have a soothing and relaxing effect on the central nervous system and skeletal muscles. Currently exercise and movement cause discomfort, therefore a review of lifestyle recommendations will occur in follow-up consultations.

Expected outcomes and follow-up protocols

Because of the extreme discomfort experienced by the patient it is predicted that compliance will be good, particularly if the initial dose provides relief. Because there are multiple health concerns (with the primary one being to resolve the gastritis), it is advisable to see the patient the following week. This will enable more medicine to be administered and the formula to be refined if necessary. Symptom improvement is expected at the follow-up consultation as long as all irritant foods, beverages and

PRESCRIPTION
Herbal formula (100 mL)

Matricaria recutita 1:2	20 mL
Filipendula ulmaria 1:2	20 mL
Calendula officinalis 1:2	15 mL
[20% EtOH]	
Tanacetum parthenium 1:5	20 mL
Glycyrrhiza glabra 1:1 HG	25 mL

Dose: 5 mL 3 × daily before food

Curcuma longa powdered extract equiv. 95% curcumin: 100 mg 3 × daily

Ulmus rubra: ½ tsp powered bark in warm water 3 × daily

Nutritional prescription

Glutamine: 2 g 3 × daily

NB: Glutamine, *Curcuma longa* and *Ulmus rubra* to be taken together in 150 mL of water 3 × daily before food

Magnesium (citrate, chelate, aspartate, orotate) 100 mg elemental magnesium per capsule:

2 capsules 2 × daily in between meals.

Lifestyle prescription

Soft diet, easily digestible, highly nutritive foods

Epsom salt baths 3 × weekly

substances are removed. It is envisaged that the herbal formula, *Ulmus rubra*, glutamine and *Curcuma longa* will be prescribed for 6–8 weeks to ensure the condition is completely resolved. A response to *Tanacetum parthenium* for migraine prophylaxis is expected to take approximately 6 weeks, although subsequent to dietary modification, with improvement in gastric symptoms coupled with central nervous system support, it is anticipated that a decrease in migraine frequency and severity will be achieved earlier. Follow-up protocols will involve further assessment of migraines, monitoring the response to *Tanacetum parthenium* and dietary, lifestyle, nutrient and herbal recommendations to improve blood glucose control.

Clinical pearls

- Focus on addressing the acute symptoms of gastritis first (in particular, pain).

- In cases of gastritis always review over-the-counter and prescription medicines to rule out causative and exacerbating factors, in this individual's case ibuprofen.

- Gastritis will present with diffuse pain, whereas an individual with a gastric ulcer will often be able to pinpoint the exact location of discomfort.

- Even though in this case food relieves symptoms, always review for changes in body weight, as this will provide insight into the pain severity and overall discomfort.

- Consider gallbladder involvement for gastritis in the absence of a *Helicobacter pylori* infection, particularly if there is also poor blood glucose control.

Expert | CONSULT

Clinical Comprehension Questions & Answers are hosted on **https://expertconsult.inkling.com/store/book/ sarris-clinical-naturopathy-case-files-1**

BIBLIOGRAPHY

Hawrelak J. Gastro-oesophageal reflux disease. In: Sarris J, Wardle J, eds. *Clinical Naturopathy: An Evidence-Based Guide to Practice*. 2nd ed. Sydney: Elsevier; 2014.

Huang X, Lv B, Zhang S, et al. Effects of radix curcumae-derived diterpenoid C on *Helicobacter pylori*-induced inflammation and nuclear factor kappa B signal pathways. *World J Gastroenterol*. 2013;19(31):5085-5931.

Schiapparelli P, Allais G, Castagnoli Gabellari I, et al. Non-pharmacological approach to migraine prophylaxis: part II. *Neurol Sci*. 2010;31(suppl 1):S137-S139.

Wider B, Pittler MH, Ernst E. Feverfew for preventing migraine. *Cochrane Database Syst Rev*. 2015;(4):CD002286.

5 | Non-alcoholic fatty liver disease

Ses Salmond

PRESENTATION

A 75-year-old woman presents with **fatigue, depression, dyspepsia**, slightly elevated alanine aminotransferase (ALT) (45 IU/L), **markedly elevated gamma-glutamyl transpeptidase** (GGT) (205 IU/L), **elevated triglycerides** (1.9 mmol/L) and **elevated glycosylated haemoglobin** (HbA$_{1C}$) (8.0%). She experienced transient ischaemic attacks about 10 years ago, a mild stroke 8 years ago and was previously diagnosed with hypothyroidism and cholelithiasis. Her current medications are thyroxine 100 mcg/day, amlodipine 10 mg/day, atorvastatin 10 mg/day and clopidogrel 75 mg/day. Her **poor diet** consists of refined carbohydrates (cakes, biscuits), excess fructose (eight pieces of fruit and 0.5 L fruit juice daily), sugar (chocolate), high dairy (cheese), minimal protein (chickpeas, lentils and nuts) and limited vegetables (peas and beans).

Diagnostic considerations

The patient has diagnosed cholelithiasis, cardiovascular disease and type 2 diabetes, which are often comorbidities in non-alcoholic fatty liver disease (NAFLD) and metabolic syndrome. The patient also presents with excess adipose tissue with a waist circumference of 88 cm, a risk factor for metabolic syndrome and NAFLD. The patient's diet of excess refined carbohydrates and a sedentary lifestyle can lead to dysglycaemia and dyslipidaemia, which may lead to free fatty acid (FFA) peroxidation, atherosclerosis and cardiovascular disease.

The biochemical picture of elevated liver enzymes (particularly ALT and GGT), raised triglycerides and dysglycaemia are highly suggestive of a diagnosis of NAFLD, particularly considering there are no risk factors for hepatitis C virus infection or alcoholic liver disease. The patient is referred back to her GP for diagnosis and for a referral to a hepatologist.

The pathogenesis of NAFLD involves the accumulation of triglycerides and lipogenesis in the liver due to insulin resistance. The consequent liver dysfunction and continued insulin resistance causes oxidative stress, driving systemic inflammation and mitochondrial dysfunction. Gut-derived endotoxaemia can exacerbate this due to poor diet.

IMPORTANT DIAGNOSTIC/CLINICAL CONSIDERATIONS

- Fatigue and depression are often comorbid with NAFLD
- Right upper-quadrant pain or discomfort or fullness possibly due to stretching of the hepatic capsule and hepatomegaly may be indicative of NAFLD
- Metabolic syndrome, diabetes mellitus, insulin resistance, hyperlipidaemia and obesity are common comorbidities. An NAFLD diagnosis may suggest these conditions or these conditions may suggest NAFLD
- Acanthosis nigricans, a cutaneous manifestation of insulin resistance, has been found in 12% of NAFLD patients. This regional hyperpigmentation is typically found in adults around the neck and over the knuckles, elbows and knees and offers clinicians and patients a physical clue as to the presence of insulin resistance

Treatment protocol

- Beneficial dietary and lifestyle changes need to be encouraged. These include prescribed regular moderate exercise (both aerobic and resistance exercises). Increased levels of quality protein (fish, soy-based protein, turkey, kangaroo, eggs, split peas) should be included as part of every meal and fibre should be increased to approximately 30 g per day (e.g. oats, psyllium, cruciferous and green leafy vegetables). Protein and fibre help with weight loss by increasing satiety. Fibre absorbs and increases the excretion of fats. A higher protein intake may reduce body weight while retaining lean body mass and supports tissue growth and repair; it is also vital to the function of the immune system.

- It is advised to reduce refined carbohydrates and fructose intake (currently eight pieces of fruit a day and 0.5 L of fruit juice) to just two pieces of fruit a day. This may reduce the dysglycaemia and lipogenesis. Inflammatory, saturated and *trans* fats in the diet can be replaced with healthy, non-inflammatory fats (e.g. replace cheese with fish such as sardines, salmon, mackerel and include flaxseeds, walnuts, avocadoes, olive oil and coconut oil).

- Encourage the use of specific medicinal foods in the diet: bitter foods such as rocket and radicchio to stimulate digestion; lecithin for membrane health; flaxseed as a source of fibre, protein, phyto-oestrogens and omega-3

FFAs; fermented foods for digestive health (e.g. yoghurt, kefir, sauerkraut and nuts and seeds for healthy snacks).

- Herbal tea therapies may be useful for increased hydration and therapeutic purposes. These include green tea for its antioxidant properties (though green tea extract should be avoided due to its potential for liver damage due to its concentrated nature). Dandelion root coffee is useful for its hepatic and cholagogue action, and mint tea can be used as a digestive aid and a substitute for carbohydrates.

- Regulation of blood glucose is needed to reduce dysglycaemia, which contributes to the metabolic syndrome picture in NAFLD due to the lipogenesis and lipolysis of FFAs with hypoglycaemics such as *Galega officinalis*, *Gymnema sylvestre*, *Silybum marianum*, *Trigonella foenum-graecum* and chromium.

- Modulate fatty acid pathways and reduce adipose tissue by increasing the excretion of FFAs via bile and increasing the beta-oxidation of FFAs with *Curcuma longa*, *Cynara scolymus*, *Silybum marianum* and vitamins D, E, coenzyme Q10 and N-acetylcysteine.

- Reduce hepatic inflammation and support optimal liver function by reducing the peroxidation of FFAs, oxidative stress and hepatic inflammation with herbal medicines and nutraceuticals with specific hepatic anti-inflammatory and antioxidant activity such as *Curcuma longa*, *Cynara scolymus*, *Silybum marianum*, *Scutellaria baicalensis*, vitamin E and N-acetylcysteine.

- Support choleretic and cholagogue function, which reduces FFAs with *Cynara scolymus*, *Silybum marianum* and *Curcuma longa*.

- Support cardiovascular health by reducing the impact of the significant comorbid factor of coronary artery disease with natural vitamin E, magnesium and coenzyme Q10.

- Support the digestive system and microbiome with *Bifidobacterium longum* and fructo-oligosaccharides as this combination has been shown to improve liver histology in non-alcoholic steatohepatitis (NASH) patients after 6 months.

Expected outcomes and follow-up protocols

In the above case, the clinical and biochemical symptom picture should improve over a 3–6-month time frame as the oxidative stress and inflammation caused by dysglycaemia and NAFLD are addressed with antioxidants, hepatoprotectives and hypoglycaemics accompanied by diet and lifestyle interventions. Monitoring biochemical results at these intervals allows the practitioner to assess the efficacy of the treatment and modify treatment as appropriate. In this case, treatment focusing

PRESCRIPTION
Herbal formula (100 mL)

Cynara scolymus 1:2	20 mL
Galega officinalis 1:2	30 mL
Gymnema sylvestre 1:2	35 mL
Trigonella foenum-graecum 1:2	15 mL

Dose: 3 mL 2 × daily before meals
Silybum marianum standardised to contain 140 mg silybin 2 × daily before meals
Curcuma longa: 1–2 tsp daily with milk or in cooking combined with black pepper

Nutritional prescription

Vitamin E (natural): 500 IU/day with meals
N-acetylcysteine: 1800 mg/day in two divided doses before meals
Magnesium: 600 mg/day with meals
Chromium: 250 mcg/day with meals
Vitamin D: 1000 IU/day with meals
Coenzyme Q10: 150 mg/day with meals

Lifestyle prescription

Avoid sugars and refined carbohydrates
Increase protein, vegetables, healthy fats and salads
Limit fruit to two pieces a day
Eat fermented foods or supplement with probiotics
Increase physical activity

on blood sugar disorders was also important—NAFLD often has comorbidities, and these must also be addressed to improve clinical and biochemical indicators of NAFLD. Failure to address comorbidities will result in not only less effective treatment of these comorbidities but also less effective treatment of NAFLD.

Clinical pearls

- A slightly elevated ALT with marked elevations in GGT and triglycerides should trigger an investigation into the presence of NAFLD.
- The ultrasound still represents the first-line diagnostic tool for simple liver steatosis (fatty liver).
- The evaluation of all NAFLD patients should consider the risks of liver disease, diabetes and cardiovascular events.

CLINICAL NATUROPATHY: IN PRACTICE

Expert | CONSULT

Clinical Comprehension Questions & Answers are hosted on
**https://expertconsult.inkling.com/store/book/
sarris-clinical-naturopathy-case-files-1**

BIBLIOGRAPHY

Cacciapuoti F, Scognamiglio A, Palumbo R, et al. Silymarin in non-alcoholic fatty liver disease. *World J Hepatol.* 2013;5:109-113.

Hernandez-Rodas MC, Valenzuela R, Videla LA. Relevant aspects of nutritional and dietary interventions in non-alcoholic fatty liver disease. *Int J Mol Sci.* 2015;16:25168-25198.

Saez-Lara MJ, Robles-Sanchez C, Ruiz-Ojeda FJ, et al. Effects of probiotics and synbiotics on obesity, insulin resistance syndrome, type 2 diabetes and non-alcoholic fatty liver disease: a review of human clinical trials. *Int J Mol Sci.* 2016;17.

Salmond SJ. Liver dysfunction and disease. In: Sarris J, Wardle J, eds. *Clinical Naturopathy: An Evidence-based Guide to Practice.* 2nd ed. Sydney: Elsevier; 2014.

Xu R, Tao A, Zhang S, et al. Association between vitamin E and non-alcoholic steatohepatitis: a meta-analysis. *Int J Clin Exp Med.* 2015;8:3924-3934.

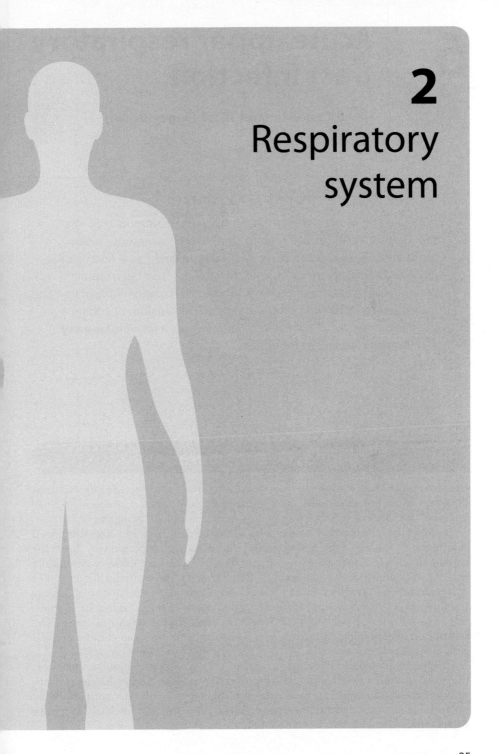

2
Respiratory system

6 | Acute upper respiratory tract infection

David Casteleijn and Tessa Finney-Brown

PRESENTATION

A 45-year-old woman presents with an **acute common cold** that she 'doesn't seem to be able to shake'. Her symptoms include **nasal catarrh, low-grade fever** and **fatigue**. She has a history of **repeated sinus infections** for which antibiotics have been regularly prescribed. She has a high-pressure job and works long hours, which causes her to suffer from **stress** and **physical tension**. In addition, she doesn't find much time to cook and so **eats a lot of take-away** and **'survives' on coffee for energy**.

Diagnostic considerations

In the common presentation above, it is not important solely to identify and treat the acute illness but to consider the contextual basis of illness. Common colds are typically viral illnesses and therefore do not require antibiotic treatment.

In this patient, her immune system may be overreacting to common viral/bacterial challenges, as evidenced by her recurrent infections and poor recovery from the current illness. This may be due to a number of factors including a chronically challenged immune system as a result of chronic stress, gastrointestinal tract (GIT) dysregulation and poor diet. Chronic sinus infections may be related to an allergy (immune hyper-responsiveness) or undertreated bacterial/fungal agents or suppression for mucus flow providing a conducive environment for various microbes. The practitioner should question the role of anatomical contributors to chronic sinusitis such as nasal polyps.

The patient presents with discomfort due to a range of acute symptoms. Therefore, the initial treatment focus should be symptomatic relief. Not only is this the patient's priority but, in meeting their needs, the practitioner will engender trust. Building upon this facet of the patient–practitioner relationship will be more likely to lead to compliance in the longer term management.

MEDICAL CONDITIONS OR SYMPTOMS THAT MAY PRESENT AS OR MIMIC ACUTE UPPER RESPIRATORY TRACT INFECTIONS

- Viral infection (common cold)
- Influenza ('the flu')
- Pneumonia
- Bronchitis
- Asthma exacerbation
- Tuberculosis (in certain parts of the world) or mycobacterial infection
- Allergies—food, environmental

Treatment protocol

- *Echinacea* spp. has immune-enhancing and immune-modulating properties. The root blend is superior in this case because the alkylamides in the *purpurea* appear to protect those in the *angustifolia* from hepatic metabolism, therefore enhancing their effect.

- *Pelargonium sidoides* is immune-enhancing and antibacterial, with research revealing significant reduction in the severity of symptoms and the duration of the common cold and sinusitis severity.

- *Euphrasia officinalis* is astringent, anticatarrhal, anti-inflammatory and a mucous membrane tonic, which makes it ideal for treating respiratory conditions with excess mucus production.

- *Sambucus nigra* (flower) has anticatarrhal and diaphoretic properties.

- *Avena sativa* (green) is included as a nerve tonic and general (but gentle) tonic because it is probable that stress is a contributing factor to her repeated infections and lowered vitality.

- *Hydrastis canadensis* is a mucous membrane trophorestorative with anticatarrhal properties, although its other antimicrobial, antibacterial and anti-inflammatory actions will also be of assistance. Unfortunately, it cannot be included in the main mixture because of the tannins in *Sambucus nigra* and *Pelargonium sidoides* (see 'Clinical pearls'). It may be prescribed as a simplex extract or tablet. Due to its endangered status, a cultivated source is recommended.

- Zinc and vitamin C are key nutrients. Zinc plays a significant role in both preventing the common cold through immune regulation and hastening recovery. While vitamin C is commonly considered a 'go-to' for the common cold, there is better evidence for its use in regulating cortisol levels and supporting the stress response (which indirectly assists in regulating the immune response). When prescribing minerals such as zinc, it is important that they be taken away from tannin-containing herbs for optimal absorption.

- Doubling the regular dose of acute remedies can be an effective temporary protocol in order to effectively treat the acute condition (assuming that the original mixture had all herbs dosed at their minimum therapeutic range, which can safely be doubled).

- It is better to dose more regularly, rather than in higher quantities, because this maintains a more consistent level of active ingredients in the body throughout the day. It also ensures optimum absorption of nutrients such as vitamin C (which is absorbed via saturable active transport).

- Because the person is acutely unwell, it is recommended that they stay home and rest. In this situation, taking herbs six times a day is not as much of an inconvenience as it would otherwise be. In this case the overall volume of herbs dispensed will need to be adjusted, simply achieved by doubling the mixture.

- Convalescence is essential. Stress to the patient that even though they may start to feel better after a day or so (depending on the severity of the acute infection) they should not go straight back to work. It is strongly recommended that she takes adequate time to recover fully. Extra sleep is likely to be required. This should be encouraged, as the patient (especially if she is stressed and busy) may not see this as a valuable use of time.

- Vegetable broths, bean and vegetable stews, rice congee and homemade chicken soup (with the whole carcass from organic chicken) provide essential immune supportive nutrients. In addition, they are psychologically comforting as traditional foods made for convalescence.

- Recommend hot lemon drinks with fresh grated ginger (and/or garlic) and raw local honey (to address an allergic rhinitis component). One traditional recipe calls for the whole lemon to be juiced (skin and all) then added to hot water with honey and brandy. Some people may find temporary relief with the addition of nutritional mucolytics to meals (e.g. grated horseradish or wasabi as a condiment).

- Hydration is important during acute illness, particularly if there is fever and resultant sweating. Moreover, when people work in high-pressure industries, or are always engaged, they can forget very simple activities such as maintaining adequate fluid intake.

PRESCRIPTION
Herbal formula (100 mL)

Echinacea root blend 1:2	20 mL
Euphrasia officinalis 1:2	20 mL
Pelargonium sidoides 1:5	20 mL
Sambucus nigra 1:2	20 mL
Avena sativa 1:2	20 mL

Dose: 5 mL every four hours in a little water or juice

Hydrastis canadensis: 500 mg tablet 3 × daily away from main mixture

Nutritional prescription

Zinc amino acid chelate: 25 mg 2 × daily away from the main mixture

Vitamin C + bioflavonoids: 1 g 3 × daily

Expected outcomes and follow-up protocols

The patient should expect improvement in acute symptoms within 2 days of beginning treatment. Full resolution should be expected within a week. Once the initial stages of illness have eased, the dose of acute herbs can be reduced to 5 mL three times each day. It is important that the initial prescription is maintained for at least a week after symptoms appear to have resolved. Therefore, follow-up with the practitioner is appropriate 1–2 weeks after the initial presentation.

Once the initial stages of illness have eased, treatment should be altered to address the predisposition to recurrent illness. Immune support should be continued but transition from an acute response to trophorestorative support with immune tonics. Adaptogens are required to enhance vitality and, in conjunction with a nervine tonic, assist bodily adaptation to stress. GIT repair is indicated here, given the background of repeated use of antibiotics, poor diet and high stress levels, all of which potentially perturb the balance of GIT flora and therefore immune responsiveness.

Herbs and nutritional supplements are important to help the patient restore a state of homeostatic balance. However, in the long term it is desirable that the patient be able to maintain a balanced and vital state through a healthy diet and lifestyle. While there are many components to an ideal diet, some foods and nutrients are particularly useful for immune function. Additionally, consider lifestyle factors such as regular exercise and sunlight—vitamin D is an essential nutrient for optimal immune function. If the patient is at risk of low vitamin D levels, these should be checked and supplementation prescribed accordingly. Consider identifying if there is underlying GIT integrity concerns and address these in the long term.

Clinical pearls

- *Hydrastis canadensis* and *Pelargonium sidoides* are not combined in one formula due to a significant interaction between the strong tannin content of *Pelargonium sidoides* and the therapeutic alkaloids of *Hydrastis canadensis*, leading to significant precipitant forming and potentially causing loss of activity of *Hydrastis canadensis* (also making the mixture very unpleasant to consume).

- Rest is critical. We can become obsessed with assisting our patients to 'soldier on' and see it as our responsibility to help them keep going to work or school rather than helping our patients understand that rest is critical and that the symptoms they are experiencing are the signs of immune activation, which deserve respect.

- Recurrent infection is not always due to an 'underactive immune system'. It is possible that the immune system is overreactive, creating an unnecessarily florid immune response (symptoms of an acute cold or rhinitis) instead of modulating the response and bringing the system back into balance with little sign of immune activation.

- Support the body and mind to combat the pathogen first, then tonify after the condition has resolved.

- Observe GIT symptoms, as dysfunction within this system may be an important contributing factor.

Expert | CONSULT

Clinical Comprehension Questions & Answers are hosted on
**https://expertconsult.inkling.com/store/book/
sarris-clinical-naturopathy-case-files-1**

BIBLIOGRAPHY

Barrett B, Brown R, Rakel D, et al. Placebo effects and the common cold: a randomized controlled trial. *Ann Fam Med.* 2011;9(4):312-322.

Casteleijn D, Finney-Brown T. Respiratory infections and immune insufficiency. In: Sarris J, Wardle J, eds. *Clinical Naturopathy: An Evidence-based Guide to Practice.* 2nd ed. Elsevier; 2014:159-182.

Cunningham-Rundles S, McNeeley DF, Moon A. Mechanisms of nutrient modulation of the immune response. *J Allergy Clin Immunol.* 2005;115(6):1119-1128.

Shah S, Sander S, White C, et al. Evaluation of echinacea for the prevention and treatment of the common cold: a meta-analysis. *Lancet Infect Dis.* 2007;7(7):347-348.

Spelman K, Burns J, Nichols D, et al. Modulation of cytokine expression by traditional medicines: a review of herbal immunomodulators. *Altern Med Rev.* 2006;11(2):128-150.

7 | Asthma

David Casteleijn and Tessa Finney-Brown

PRESENTATION

A 46-year-old male presents with a recent diagnosis and onset of **asthma**. He is currently taking inhaled corticosteroids and bronchodilators. His asthma is **made worse by aspirin, certain food additives and stress**. In addition he **suffers from indigestion and heartburn**.

Diagnostic considerations

This patient's asthma appears to have an atopic basis because it has associations with aspirin and food additives. Allergy is associated with an exaggerated inflammatory immune response, which provokes the release of additional inflammatory mediators (e.g. histamine and platelet-activating factor (PAF)), intensifying initial bronchoconstriction.

To address this facet of the presentation, it is essential to modulate the immune response and dampen the inflammatory cascade as well as identifying and treating the cause of the heightened immune response if possible. Stress has been demonstrated to cause significant exacerbation of inflammation, therefore addressing the patient's heightened stress response is an important objective here.

A clear connection between digestive dysfunction and bronchoconstriction has been demonstrated. Additionally, there is the more involved naturopathic understanding that chronic digestive dysregulation often contributes to immune dysregulation and predisposes the patient to allergies (refer to the digestive system chapters). While the above actions will ease asthmatic flare-ups, direct symptom relief is also required, and to this end specific bronchodilators need to be prescribed.

Treatment protocol

Asthma is one condition in which many herbal medicines have specific targeted actions.

> **MEDICAL CONDITIONS OR SYMPTOMS THAT MAY MIMIC ASTHMA**
> - Chronic obstructive pulmonary disease (wheeze, cough—usually productive)
> - Bronchiectasis (cough)
> - Lung cancer (cough, chest symptoms)
> - Postnasal drip (cough)
> - Allergic reaction (chest tightness and wheeze)
> - Gastro-oesophageal reflux (chronic cough)
> - Medications (e.g. ACE inhibitor) (chronic cough)
> - Anxiety disorders (anxiety response affecting respiration)

- *Albizia lebbeck* is included in the formula due to its antiallergenic properties and demonstrated specific effectiveness in asthma of recent (less than 2 years) diagnosis.
- *Adhatoda vasica* and *Euphorbia* spp. exhibit substantial bronchodilator properties.
- *Pelargonium sidoides* is immune modulating and antibacterial, with research showing significantly less frequent asthma attacks and shortening of respiratory infections.
- *Glycyrrhiza glabra* is a soothing demulcent employed to treat the mucous membranes and, as a result, a secondary antitussive. *Glycyrrhiza glabra* is also adaptogenic and an 'adrenal tonic', and will support the patient through his times of stress.
- *Gentiana lutea* is a strong bitter, included due to its beneficial effect on digestive irregularities.
- *Zingiber officinale* also provides general digestive support and helps compensate for the traditional 'cooling' effect that bitters like *Gentiana lutea* can have on digestion.
- *Boswellia serrata* has supportive evidence in treating asthma by exerting an anti-inflammatory activity, which is synergistically enhanced by its combination with *Curcuma longa* and *Zingiber officinale,* both of which are also demonstrated anti-inflammatories. Due to its nature as a resin, *Boswellia serrata* is not ideally administered in extract form, hence its prescription in tablet form.
- Magnesium is included for its muscle relaxing properties, using a combination of forms to enhance absorption and bioavailability. Doses at the higher end of the supplementary range are recommended in the initial stage of treatment in order to overcome any potential chronic deficiency (assessed

via a blood test or the diet). The dose will be reduced as the treatment phase moves from acute response to long-term management.

- Omega-3 fatty acids are included due to marked anti-inflammatory effects and can also be found from foods.
- Quercetin reduces inflammation and may acutely relax airway smooth muscle.

Herbs and nutritional supplements are important in helping the patient to restore a state of homeostatic balance. However, it is desirable that the patient be able to maintain a balanced and vital state through healthy dietary and lifestyle choices. Recognising that there are many components to an ideal diet, some foods and nutrients are particularly useful for immune function in asthma. These include foods with antimicrobial compounds (garlic, onions and shallots) and foods rich in vitamins A, C and E because diets high in fruit and vegetables have been demonstrated to reduce the risk of wheeze and asthma in both adults and children.

PRESCRIPTION
Herbal formula (100 mL)

Albizia lebbeck 1:2	25 mL
Pelargonium sidoides 1:5	25 mL
Glycyrrhiza glabra 1:1	15 mL
Adhatoda vasica 1:2	15 mL
Euphorbia spp. 1:2	10 mL
Gentiana lutea 1:2	5 mL
Zingiber officinale 1:2	5 mL

Dose: 5 mL 3 × daily before meals

Herbal tablet

Boswellia serrata: 2 g
Curcuma longa: 2 g
Zingiber officinale: 300 mg
combined in tablet form
2 tablets 3 × daily

Nutritional prescription

Magnesium orotate/citrate combination: 400 mg 2 × daily
Omega-3 fatty acids: 3.2 g EPA/day; 2.2 g DHA/day

Expected outcomes and follow-up protocols

The above prescription should produce significant improvements within days. It is suggested that this treatment be maintained for a number of weeks.

Once the patient appears stable, treatment can move towards addressing the underlying causes of the condition. These may be considered to include chronic immune dysregulation in part as a result of long-term gastrointestinal dysbiosis and, potentially, increased gut permeability. Herbs such as *Hydrastis canadensis* can be added to enhance gastrointestinal tract repair, or general or nervous tonics or nutritives such as *Astragalus membranaceus* or *Avena sativa* can be used. *Ginkgo biloba* could also be considered with its anti-PAF action as another way to break the inflammatory cycle feeding itself.

Clinical pearls

- It is critically important to ensure any patient with an acute asthma presentation is aware that, despite the inclusion of 'bronchodilators', their herbal mixture is not a direct replacement for medically prescribed treatments, which need to be continued until reviewed by their medical practitioner.

- Controlling inflammation is central—it is essential to identify what is driving the chronic immune activation/inflammation and address this if long-term change is to be effected.

- *Ginkgo biloba* is commonly thought to affect clotting because it inhibits PAF; however, PAF is much more important as an inflammatory mediator than in blood clotting.

- *Hydrastis canadensis* and *Pelargonium sidoides* are not combined in the one formula due to a significant interaction between the strong tannin content of *Pelargonium sidoides* and the therapeutic alkaloids of *Hydrastis canadensis*, leading to significant precipitant forming and potentially causing loss of activity of *Hydrastis canadensis* (making the mixture unpleasant to consume).

Expert | CONSULT

Clinical Comprehension Questions & Answers are hosted on
**https://expertconsult.inkling.com/store/book/
sarris-clinical-naturopathy-case-files-1**

BIBLIOGRAPHY

Borchers AT, Selmi C, Meyers FJ, et al. Probiotics and immunity. *J Gastroenterol.* 2009;44(1):26-46.

Casteleijn D, Finney-Brown T. Asthma. In: Sarris J, Wardle J, eds. *Clinical Naturopathy: An Evidence-Based Guide to Practice.* 2nd ed. Elsevier; 2014:183-204.

Mali R, Dhake A. A review on herbal antiasthmatics. *Orient Pharm Exp Med.* 2011;11(2):77-90.

Mickleborough TD. A nutritional approach to managing exercise-induced asthma. *Exerc Sport Sci Rev.* 2008;36(3):135-144.

von Mutius E, Braun-Fahrländer C, Schierl R, et al. Exposure to endotoxin or other bacterial components might protect against the development of atopy. *Clin Exp Allergy.* 2000;30(9):1230-1234.

8 Chronic sinusitis

David Casteleijn and Tessa Finney-Brown

PRESENTATION

A 32-year-old male presents with **constant nasal congestion** and **sinus pressure**, which 'comes and goes' in severity but has been ongoing for at least 2 years. The pressure and associated facial pain are **aggravated by bending over or lying down**, with an **underlying dull headache**. During **acute flare-ups nasal discharge is thick and yellow-coloured**. The patient has a **history of regular prescriptions of antibiotics** and **use of antihistamines**.

Diagnostic considerations

The primary aim is to aid the removal of congested mucus, which acts as a reservoir for infection. The patient will need to agree to, and be fully informed about, this process because there is likely to be a period of increased discomfort as the mucus is liquefied and expelled.

A key priority is to help the patient avoid the use of antihistamines, as many practitioners feel these may prevent the long-term resolution of the condition by drying up the secretions (therefore maintaining a pathogenic reservoir).

The patient also requires immune support and antimicrobials. Once the acute infection has eased, long-term management will need to address the underlying causes of immune dysregulation, potentially influenced by altered colonic microflora, unhealthy lifestyle choices and increased gastrointestinal tract permeability. If sinus congestion has been ongoing for many years, it is recommended that the patient be referred to a medical practitioner to exclude anatomical idiosyncrasies that inhibit free drainage of mucus.

Treatment protocol

- A hot *Trigonella foenum-graecum* infusion taken 3 × daily. Raw honey can be added to assist with taste if needed. This may be made by steeping 10 g of fenugreek seeds in boiling water for 5 minutes. Alternatively, 5 mL of

> **MEDICAL CONDITIONS OR SYMPTOMS THAT MAY APPEAR AS OR EXACERBATE CHRONIC SINUSITIS**
> - Infection—viral, bacterial, fungal
> - Allergic rhinitis
> - Vasomotor rhinitis
> - Food allergy/intolerance symptoms
> - Nasal polyp
> - Nasal tumour

the herbal extract can be added to boiling water. The mucolytic activity will liquefy mucosal secretions to clear the nasal passages, removing the reservoir for chronic infection.

- *Echinacea* root blend (60/40 *purpurea/angustifolia*) was chosen for its immune modulating properties. It assists in regulating a potentially over-responsive immune system, being astringent, anticatarrhal, anti-inflammatory and a mucous membrane tonic.
- *Euphrasia officinalis* is particularly useful to control the excess production of mucus.
- *Foeniculum vulgare* synergistically enhances the mucolytic action of *Trigonella foenum-graecum*, clearing congestion and removing the microbial reservoir. Additionally, it addresses infection directly, via its antibacterial action.
- *Pelargonium sidoides* is beneficial for use in rhinosinusitis, reducing the symptoms and enhancing resolution of the condition. It is antimicrobial and a marked immune modulator.
- *Albizia lebbeck* is antiallergic to alleviate the immediate symptoms and also reduce the need for antihistamine medication.
- Betacarotene, a vitamin A precursor and antioxidant, helps repair damaged cells of the mucous membranes. It also reduces membrane sensitivity to various irritants.
- Papain and pancreatin digest mucus accumulations, break up immune complexes and provide anti-inflammatory activity. Combined with the mucolytic garlic, this combination is effective at breaking down sinus congestion.
- The patient should be advised to maintain or increase fluid intake to assist with hydration of the mucous membranes. In the case of any acute infection, it is important to rest and avoid excess stress in order to enhance the body's healing capacity.

- Onions, garlic and shallots can be emphasised in the diet, as they have strong antimicrobial activity. Garlic in particular needs to be used raw, but if used in cooking, heat it for less than 5 minutes where possible to preserve the active constituent (*allicin*). Shallots, however, appear to retain their antimicrobial activity after significant heating for long periods.

- Chicken soup has also demonstrated mucolytic and antimicrobial properties and is an easy way to encourage increased fluid intake.

- Known allergenic foods should be avoided. Some practitioners may wish to advise the avoidance of foods that are commonly considered 'mucus causing' or inflammatory (e.g. wheat, dairy and sugar), but there is weak scientific evidence to support this.

- The use of nasal irrigation (hypertonic saline with a neti pot or nasal rinse) may assist in clearing chronic infection and preventing further acute exacerbations of sinusitis. The high osmotic pull of hypertonic saline acts to increase fluid in the nasal passages, encouraging clearance of congested mucus.

PRESCRIPTION
Herbal formula (100 mL)

Echinacea root blend 1:2	20 mL
Euphrasia officinalis 1:2	20 mL
Foeniculum vulgare 1:2	15 mL
Pelargonium sidoides 1:5	20 mL
Albizia lebbeck 1:2	25 mL

Dose: 5 mL 3 × daily in a little water or juice

Herbal infusion

Trigonella foenum-graecum 10 g as a hot infusion 3 × daily

Nutritional prescription
Tablet formula 1:

Betacarotene: 1500 IU
Vitamin D3: 150–200 IU
Papain: 60 mg
2 tablets 3 × daily during the initial stage of treatment

Tablet formula 2:

Allium sativum equivalent to fresh bulb: 3.6 g
1 tablet 2 × daily during the initial stage of treatment

- It is important to educate the patient on the effects of the medication they may use for the condition. Unnecessary antibiotic overuse may lead to gastrointestinal dysbiosis, and while antihistamines reduce nasal symptoms they may contribute to chronicity of a condition. That said, there is a time and place for these medications, and the patient should be advised to weigh up the pros and cons in each situation.

Expected outcomes and follow-up protocols

The above prescription should produce a significant improvement within days. It is suggested that this treatment be maintained for a number of weeks. Many of the suggested treatments, especially dietary changes, may be beneficial in the long term. Once the symptoms have stabilised, treatment can move towards addressing the underlying causes of the condition, which are similar to those for asthma, as they include chronic immune dysregulation as a result of long-term gastrointestinal dysbiosis and, potentially, increased gut permeability (see gastrointestinal system cases).

Clinical pearls

- Central to both the acute and the ongoing treatment of chronic sinusitis is the removal of the reservoir harbouring the microbes that led to the infection and contribute to the ongoing inflammation.

- It is critical to identify what is driving the chronic immune activation/inflammation and address this if long-term change is to be effected.

- Where possible the patient can be encouraged to avoid antihistamines as there is a theory that the extreme drying effect can exacerbate congestion.

Expert|CONSULT

Clinical Comprehension Questions & Answers are hosted on
**https://expertconsult.inkling.com/store/book/
sarris-clinical-naturopathy-case-files-1**

BIBLIOGRAPHY

Casteleijn D, Finney-Brown T. Sarris J, Wardle J, eds. 'Congestive respiratory disorders', *Clinical Naturopathy: An Evidence-Based Guide to Practice E2*. Elsevier; 2014:205-223.

Guo R, Canter PH, Ernst E. Herbal medicines for the treatment of rhinosinusitis: a systematic review. *Otolaryngol Head Neck Surg*. 2006;135(4):496-506.

Lim M, Citardi MJ, Leong JL. Topical antimicrobials in the management of chronic rhinosinusitis: a systematic review. *Am J Rhinol*. 2008;22(4):381-389.

Sadowska AM, Manuel YKB, De Backer WA. Antioxidant and anti-inflammatory efficacy of NAC in the treatment of COPD: discordant in vitro and in vivo dose-effects: a review. *Pulm Pharmacol Ther*. 2007;20(1):9-22.

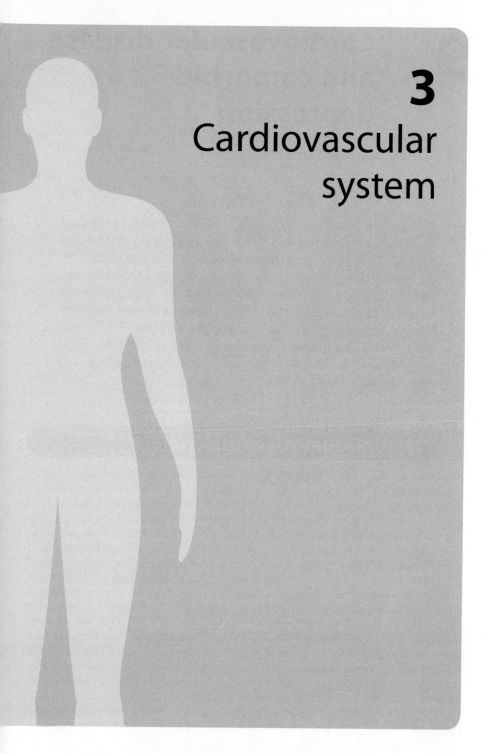

3
Cardiovascular system

9 Cardiovascular disease and comorbid depression

Jerome Sarris

PRESENTATION

A 62-year-old male is seeking treatment options after being diagnosed with **atherosclerosis** via an angiography and stress testing. He was also diagnosed with **high cholesterol** after a blood test: triglycerides (fasting) 2.0, total cholesterol 7.1 mmol/L, HDL 2.0 mmol/L and LDL 4.2 mmol/L. He is not obese and is a non-smoker; however, he reveals regular consumption of **high levels of alcohol and fatty food**, in addition to leading a **sedentary lifestyle**. The patient reports occasional **depressive episodes**. He has felt that his mood has been getting lower over the past couple of weeks (4/10), and **feels very cold**. He is currently taking low-dose statin medication.

Diagnostic considerations

The initial consideration is for the clinician to have a firm understanding of cardiovascular disease (CVD) and the impact it may have on a range of systems. Atherosclerosis affects various regions of the circulation and will present with unique clinical symptoms depending on which arteries are affected. In coronary arteries it causes myocardial infarction and angina, whereas stroke and transient cerebral ischaemia can occur when it is present in the arteries of the nervous system. Atherogenesis or the pathogenesis of atherosclerosis usually occurs over decades. The eventual clinical manifestation may be chronic, as is the case in angina, or acute, such as a heart attack or stroke or sudden death. Regardless, individuals may live with atherosclerosis and experience no symptoms or reduced life expectancy and morbidity. Cardiovascular risk is positively associated with low-density lipoprotein (LDL-C) levels and inversely with high-density lipoprotein (HDL-C) levels. Blood levels of lipoprotein(a) have also been found to have an association with cardiovascular risk. The relationship between fasting serum triglyceride (TG) and cardiovascular risk is confounded by the inverse association between TG and HDL-C, as well as by the association of TG with other risk factors such as diabetes mellitus and body mass.

Due to these elements, it is critical for the clinician to assist in managing the lipid profile, in addition to appreciating the potential impact of the future development of metabolic issues. In the above case, while the patient is not obese, that does not mean that metabolic issues are not present. Therefore, check biomarkers of risk, such as resting blood sugar levels. Depression is a common precursor to CVD and, because his depression is ongoing, this will need to be addressed. One of the key intersecting pathophysiological elements between CVD and depression is inflammation, therefore the use of anti-inflammatory interventions will be beneficial.

IMPORTANT CLINICAL CONSIDERATIONS

- A thorough case history is needed, especially in respect to family history of CVD
- Blood tests, medical tests and appropriate referral are required
- Depression is commonly comorbid with CVD; each increases the risk of the other
- An integrative approach focusing on lifestyle changes, medical/ nutraceutical intervention and psychological techniques may be of benefit

Treatment protocol

- Aside from judicious nutraceutical prescription, lifestyle modification is at the core of the above patient's naturopathic treatment. As a minimum, give all patients dietary advice. This includes enriching their diet with a good source of fibre, both soluble and insoluble, between 10 and 60 g daily. A lower refined carbohydrate diet may assist in alterations in fatty acid composition and reduced inflammation compared with a low-fat diet, in addition to reducing atherosclerosis. A diet high in prebiotic and probiotic foods may beneficially influence the microbiome, which in turn may reduce inflammation and therefore have a positive effect on brain and cardiovascular health.
- The patient should reduce his alcohol intake to a low or moderate level (e.g. one or two glasses of red wine a few times a week). Binge drinking, particularly with beer and spirits, should be gently discouraged.
- Advise the patient to increase activity and begin a graded exercise plan with medical approval. The optimal level of exercise is the equivalent of 20–40 minutes daily approximately 5 days per week, of an intensity at 65–80% peak oxygen consumption. It should, however, be noted that even lesser duration with bursts of high intensity may also be of benefit.
- Herbal treatments focus on a range of actions to benefit cardiovascular integrity and function, and to improve mood. *Cynara scolymus* is beneficial

as an antioxidant and choleretic. It reduces the oxidative effects on plasma lipids at the same time as reducing their levels. *Allium sativum* is beneficial for both its antithrombotic activity and its ability to modify lipid components, as well as in raising HDL-C levels and reducing both TG and LDL-C fractions in the blood. *Crataegus oxyacantha* possesses many cardiovascular benefits, particularly the ability to reduce resting diastolic blood pressure and heart rate as well as potent antioxidant activity.

- *Rhodiola rosea* is a mood elevator, adaptogenic and cardiotonic. *Rosmarinus officinalis* is a traditional 'stimulating cerebral tonic', having potentially beneficial antioxidant properties. It is also a warming circulatory stimulant that may benefit his 'feeling of coldness'. This action is fortified by *Zingiber officinale* as an anti-inflammatory and circulatory stimulant.

- Coenzyme Q10 has a positive effect in reducing oxidative stress, as well as other antiatherogenic effects. Prescribe fish oil (standardised for higher eicosapentaenoic acid or 'EPA') to modify plasma lipid profiles and increase HDL-C levels while reducing LDL-C and TG fractions. Its ability to reduce platelet aggregation makes it particularly good for patients at risk of infarction and stroke.

PRESCRIPTION
Herbal formula (100 mL)

Cynara scolymus 1:2	30 mL
Crataegus oxyacantha 1:1	25 mL
Rhodiola rosea 2:1	20 mL
Rosmarinus officinalis 2:1	20 mL
Zingiber officinale 2:1	5 mL

Dose: 5 mL 3 × daily
Allium sativum capsules: 2 g 2 × daily

Nutritional prescription

Co-Q10: 150 mg daily
Omega-3 fish oil (equivalent to approximately 1 g of EPA per day)

Lifestyle prescription

Moderate balanced exercise
Sleep hygiene
Mindfulness meditation
Dietary improvement

Expected outcomes and follow-up protocols

In treating a patient with atherosclerosis, the aim is to minimise or prevent the long-term sequelae of the condition. Assess patients for both their cardiovascular risk and their treatment benefit. It is prudent to encourage high-risk patients to seek medical advice immediately and consider pharmaceutical intervention or treatment modification (if the naturopathic prescription does not beneficially alter the biomarkers after 2–3 months).

Give all patients of varying risk levels dietary advice; however, see obese patients weekly and give strict dietary guidelines with the aim to reducing their weight by at least 2 kg monthly. Consider plant sterols as another therapeutic option in reducing the more harmful blood fat fractions such as LDL-C, TG and total cholesterol; however, note that the evidence underpinning this has been questioned. *Curcuma longa* is another potential option as it may provide anti-inflammatory, cardiovascular-protective and antidepressant effects.

Consider seeing non-obese patients fortnightly for the first month to work out any treatment problems, and then monthly, since body and blood changes take months to occur. Routinely perform blood pressure readings at each visit. The only way to clinically determine therapeutic outcomes with atherosclerosis is through blood examination, which ideally should be performed every 6 months. So it is best to work with the patient and their medical practitioner. Referring the patient for a lipoprotein(a) test may also be of benefit in determining cardiovascular risk.

Monitor his mood, which is expected to improve over the course of weeks. If no improvement has occurred (or if it has worsened), he may need to be appropriately referred. Note that there can be some metabolic consequences of commencing antidepressants, and therefore careful consideration is needed if this therapeutic approach is being considered. A final comment is that *Zingiber officinale* and *Rosmarinus officinalis* tend to be fairly acrid tasting, and therefore tolerance may need to be considered.

Clinical pearls

- Atherosclerosis and dyslipidaemia are chronic conditions that need to be consistently treated.

- Small changes in blood lipid levels may have significant effects on health.

- Consider the effect of comorbidities on cardiovascular health, in particular clinical depression.

- Blood-test monitoring may assist in assessing treatment outcomes.

Expert | CONSULT

Clinical Comprehension Questions & Answers are hosted on
**https://expertconsult.inkling.com/store/book/
sarris-clinical-naturopathy-case-files-1**

Acknowledgement

This case has been modified from Michael Alexander's case study in the first edition of *Clinical Naturopathy*.

BIBLIOGRAPHY

Alexander M. Atherosclerosis and dyslipidaemia. In: Sarris and Wardle, ed. *Clinical Naturopathy: An Evidence-Based Guide to Practice*. Sydney: Elsevier; 2010.

Dhar AK, Barton DA. Depression and the link with cardiovascular disease. *Front Psychiatry*. 2016;7:33.

Ghasemian M, Owlia S, Owlia MB. Review of anti-inflammatory herbal medicines. *Adv Pharmacol Sci*. 2016.

O'Neil A, Williams ED, Stevenson CE, et al. Co-morbid cardiovascular disease and depression: sequence of disease onset is linked to mental but not physical self-rated health. Results from a cross-sectional, population-based study. *Soc Psychiatry Psychiatr Epidemiol*. 2012;47(7):1145-1151.

Topol EJ, Califf RM, Prystowsky EN, et al. *Textbook of Cardiovascular Medicine*. 3rd ed. Lippincott Williams & Wilkins; 2007.

10 | Hypertension

Jon Wardle

PRESENTATION

A 53-year-old overweight male patient presents to the clinic after a diagnosis with **hypertension**. He originally saw his doctor because he had **dizziness** on and off for several weeks with **headache** and **fatigue** that he thought was an infection. An electrocardiogram (ECG) has revealed that he also has **slight left ventricular hypertrophy**. He has concerns because **his father died of a stroke when he was 49**. He is also a social smoker.

Diagnostic considerations

Hypertension is a *sustained* rise in *resting* blood pressure (BP). It is important to accurately measure blood pressure by sphygmomanometry—usually over three consecutive visits—as readings can be confounded by some clinically pertinent conditions. This includes 'masked' hypertension (where normotensive readings are observed in the clinic but hypertensive readings occur at home) and 'white coat' hypertension (where anxiety during a clinic visit can result in artificially raised BP). Most people (approximately 90%) have primary or essential (no known cause) hypertension. Secondary hypertension (where there is a known cause) is most likely to be the result of kidney disease but can also be caused by coarctation of the aorta, endocrine disease and pregnancy. Left ventricular hypertrophy usually develops in response to some factor, such as high BP, that requires the left ventricle to work harder. As the workload increases, the walls of the chamber grow thicker, lose elasticity and eventually may fail to pump with as much force as a healthy heart. Left ventricular hypertrophy presents with increased risk of heart disease including heart attack, heart failure, irregular heartbeats (arrhythmia) and sudden cardiac arrest. It also suggests a longstanding issue with BP in this patient.

A naturopathic approach to hypertension doesn't simply categorise hypertension as primary or idiopathic, but assumes that there exists a definite cause–effect relationship, even in primary (idiopathic) hypertension. Differing hypertension prevalence among certain population and age groups is partially due to differences in the intake of certain nutrients. Sustained raised BP is positively associated with higher sodium, alcohol and protein intakes, and is inversely associated with potassium, calcium and

45

magnesium intake. Increased homocysteine levels are also associated with various cardiovascular conditions. Due to this, dietary and lifestyle measures are of primary focus in treating hypertension. Hypertension rarely exists without other comorbidities, so investigation for other health issues is also necessary.

SYMPTOMS THAT MAY BE ASSOCIATED WITH OR AGGRAVATE (PRIMARY) HYPERTENSION

- Renal artery or vascular disease or aortic coarctation
- Unexplained hypokalaemia
- Phaeochromocytoma
- Abdominal/lumbar trauma
- Kidney disease—chronic glomerulonephritis, pyelonephritis, obstructive nephropathy
- Medication-induced hypertension (e.g. birth control pills)
- Endocrine diseases such as Cushing's disease
- Psychiatric disorders (anxiety/stress disorders)

Treatment protocol

- The focus of the herbal formula is to exert a hypotensive action via smooth muscle relaxation, vasodilation and stress reduction (*Valeriana* spp. and *Crataegus oxyacantha*). A diuretic effect may occur via *Taraxacum officinale*, which can result in lower blood pressure (and is the mechanism of action of many conventional hypertension medications). *Ginkgo biloba* may be of benefit in improving circulation and enhancing vascular integrity.

- Fish oil rich in docosahexaenoic acid (DHA) can be taken at a dose of six capsules daily (1000 mg fish oil per capsule) to increase arterial elasticity. Magnesium also indirectly produces vasodilation. Vitamin B6 in a daily dose of 100 mg and vitamin B12 in a dose of 1000 mcg daily will assist healthy homocysteine metabolism. It may be appropriate to use a sublingual form of B12 to overcome the low levels of intrinsic factor that may preclude gut absorption. Folic acid can be taken in a daily dose of 500 mcg. *Allium sativum* can also be prescribed or increased in the diet to augment the hypotensive action of the prescription, using methods that improve or increase compliance (e.g. roasted if raw cannot be tolerated).

- Dietary and lifestyle modifications should be introduced because these are essential in reducing the risk factors associated with hypertension. The Mediterranean diet is recommended because it provides a convenient and accessible way for this patient to increase fruit and vegetable intake and to eat meat products with healthier fat profiles.

- There is strong epidemiological and experimental evidence to support a positive link between the lowering of BP and exercise. Aerobic exercise that uses large muscle groups for 20–60 minutes a day for a minimum of 3 days a week is advisable. Strength training has also been shown to reduce arterial blood pressure and is advised. Due to the history of serious cardiovascular morbidity in this patient's family history these exercises should be gradually introduced over time.
- As stress and anxiety can exacerbate hypertension, stress-reduction exercises and interventions are encouraged, as well as interventions to improve sleep.

PRESCRIPTION
Herbal formula (100 mL)

Valeriana officinalis 1:2	25 mL
Crataegus oxyacantha 1:2	25 mL
Ginkgo biloba 2:1	25 mL
Taraxacum officinale leaf 1:2	25 mL
Dose: 7 mL 2 × daily	

Nutritional prescription

Magnesium chelate: 200 mg 2 × daily
(400 mg elemental mg daily)
Omega-3 fish oil (1:1 EPA:DHA ratio): 3 g 2 × daily
Vitamin B2, B6, B5 100 mg of each daily
Folic acid: 500 mcg/B12 1000 mcg 1 × daily

Lifestyle prescription

Moderate balanced exercise
Sleep hygiene and mindfulness meditation
Dietary improvement (including a Mediterranean diet, raw/pressed/roasted garlic and a reduction in carbohydrates for cardiovascular health, and general dietary counselling)

Expected outcomes and follow-up protocols

The outcomes affecting future protocols can be broadly divided into two groups: those that are objective (measurable) and those that are subjective. The measurable outcomes that have the greatest influence on the treatment regimen are:

- weight and body mass index
- blood pressure (it is recommended that the patient buys a basic automated blood pressure monitor and this should be augmented with BP and pulse readings at each consultation)

- full blood examination, which should provide information about other risk factors that should be considered in all vascular disease (blood lipids, insulin levels, etc.).

Patients with hypertension rarely present without other comorbidities, and may bring with them a history of other therapy and practitioner use. The patient in this case is already in contact with a medical practitioner and, given his family history, it would be prudent to ensure he maintains this contact and has regular blood test reviews, which are shared with all his practitioners. This is especially important since he is overweight and has a family history of stroke, which is usually associated with dyslipidaemia. The patient is strongly advised to reduce his weight to a healthier level and stop smoking. He also needs to adopt an exercise program, which will have beneficial effects on both his weight and his stress.

Of the subjective outcomes, those associated with satisfaction of treatment and reduction in stress, as well as with feelings of empowerment, are the most significant to take note of. After an initial consultation it would then be prudent to have a weekly follow-up for a month, then fortnightly return visits for another month, then four more monthly visits. At this 6-month point of treatment, if there are encouraging signs that there has been significant weight loss (assume an average of 0.5–1 kg/month) and adequate blood pressure control (BP ≤ 130/80 in ≥ 80% of monitor readings), then follow-up consultations could be extended to 6-monthly.

Clinical pearls

- Make treatment decisions based on long-term maintenance of this condition.
- Treatment with prescribed medicines (natural or pharmaceutical) is not enough; dietary and lifestyle changes are essential.
- Other comorbid conditions may exist that exacerbate hypertension, so be sure to examine these as part of your treatment
- Exercise in patients with cardiovascular diseases should be implemented in a graded fashion, preferably under the guidance of a health practitioner.
- Blood pressure monitoring by the patient is itself an important aspect of treatment.

Expert|CONSULT

Clinical Comprehension Questions & Answers are hosted on **https://expertconsult.inkling.com/store/book/ sarris-clinical-naturopathy-case-files-1**

Acknowledgement
This case has been modified from Michael Alexander's case study in the first edition of *Clinical Naturopathy*.

BIBLIOGRAPHY
Alexander M. Hypertension and stroke. In: Sarris J, Wardle J, eds. *Clinical Naturopathy: An Evidence-Based Guide to Practice*. Sydney: Churchill Livingstone; 2010.

Dibona G. Sympathetic nervous system and hypertension. *Hypertens*. 2013;61(3):556-560.

Levine GN. *Cardiology Secrets*. 3rd ed. Philadelphia: Saunders; 2010:285-292.

Pase MP, Grima NA, Sarris J. The effects of dietary and nutrient interventions on arterial stiffness. *Am J Clin Nutr*. 2011;93:446-454.

Zhao JG, Cao CH, Liu CZ, et al. Effect of acupuncture treatment on spastic states of stroke patients. *J Neurol Sci*. 2009;276(1-2):143-147.

11 | Erectile dysfunction

Matthew Leach

PRESENTATION

A 55-year-old male presents with **erectile dysfunction** and **lack of libido** for the past 6 months. The man is **obese** (BMI = 30.2 kg/m²), **hypertensive** (150/95 mmHg), a social **drinker** and a social **smoker**, and has a history of **sleep apnoea, hypercholesterolaemia** (6.7 mmol/L) and **hypertriglyceridaemia** (2.0 mmol/L). His **diet is poor**, containing high levels of refined carbohydrates and low levels of fibre, fruit and vegetables.

Diagnostic considerations

The aetiology of erectile dysfunction (ED) is often multifactorial. As such, it is critical that any person presenting with ED undergoes a comprehensive health history and physical examination and that all contributing factors are identified prior to planning treatment. Psychogenic factors, such as performance anxiety, depression and post-traumatic stress disorder, can be a cause, though are often uncommon relative to other causes. Organic disease can often contribute to ED, including cardiovascular disease (e.g. hypertension or dyslipidaemia), respiratory conditions (e.g. sleep apnoea), endocrine disease (e.g. diabetes mellitus or hyperthyroidism) and neurological disorders (e.g. neuropathy or temporal lobe epilepsy), many of which are present in this case. ED is also a common adverse effect of several medications, including antihypertensives, antidepressants, antipsychotics and antiulcerants. Iatrogenic causes, such as radiotherapy and pelvic surgery, can also be responsible. As ED can be a manifestation of serious disease (such as renal failure and liver cirrhosis), medical referral is strongly advised in order to rule out any such conditions.

**SYMPTOMS THAT MAY BE ASSOCIATED WITH
OR AGGRAVATE ERECTILE DYSFUNCTION**

- Cardiovascular disorders
- Stress and anxiety
- Fatigue levels
- Psychological factors
- Metabolic issues
- Nerve damage
- Medication side effects

Treatment protocol

- ED is now considered a key indicator for cardiovascular assessment in men. The underlying cause of ED in this case is likely to be cardiovascular disease (i.e. hypertension and dyslipidaemia) and, as such, is the focus of treatment.

- Meditation can be encouraged because it has been shown to produce clinically meaningful reductions in both systolic and diastolic blood pressure.

- Dietary advice is essential, especially guidance on increasing fruit and vegetable intake and replacing refined carbohydrates with wholegrain foods, as dietary advice can bring about modest improvements in blood pressure and total and low-density lipoprotein (LDL) cholesterol.

- Smoking is an independent risk factor for hypertension and ED; guidance on the cessation of smoking is therefore strongly advised.

- *Valeriana officinalis* extract is added to the herbal formulation as it demonstrates anxiolytic, antihypertensive and anticoronaryspastic activity in vivo. *Crataegus oxyacantha* has been shown to reduce resting diastolic blood pressure in mildly hypertensive subjects. *Cynara scolymus* may reduce serum cholesterol levels in patients with hypercholesterolaemia. *Taraxacum officinale* root and leaf has been shown in animal models to improve plasma antioxidant enzyme activity and lipid profiles.

- Magnesium hydroxide has been shown to produce modest reductions in total cholesterol in healthy subjects and small reductions in diastolic blood pressure in adults with primary hypertension.

- Omega-3 polyunsaturated fatty acid supplementation generates clinically significant improvements in blood triglyceride levels in adults with cardiovascular risk factors.

PRESCRIPTION
Herbal formula (100 mL)

Valeriana officinalis 1:2	25 mL
Crataegus oxyacantha 1:2	25 mL
Cynara scolymus 2:1	25 mL
Taraxacum officinale 2:1	25 mL
Dose: 7 mL 2 × daily	

Nutritional prescription

Magnesium hydroxide: 200 mg 2 × daily
Omega-3 fish oil: 3 g 2 × daily

Lifestyle prescription

Moderate balanced exercise
Smoking cessation
Transcendental meditation
Dietary modification

Expected outcomes and follow-up protocols

Dietary and lifestyle modification, which are important elements of any treatment plan for cardiovascular disease, can be difficult to maintain for some people. Providing clear, achievable and realistic goals, emotional support, suitable educational aids and regular review and follow-up may help with improving concordance with treatment.

The effectiveness of the treatment plan can be monitored through regular assessments of blood pressure, weight, diet, exercise and smoking status (e.g. at least monthly), and measurement of blood lipids (e.g. at least every 6 months). If the treatment plan is followed as advised, the patient may expect to lose approximately 1 kg of body weight per week; a reduction in the patient's BMI from 30.2 kg/m^2 (obese) to < 25 kg/m^2 (normal weight) would translate to an 18 kg weight loss over 18 weeks. The treatment regimen may also see blood pressure fall to under 130/80 mmHg within 6 months, and serum cholesterol reduce to under 5.5 mmol/L within 12 months. Notable improvements in ED would be expected to transpire within a year. If the patient can sustain the treatment in the long term, then other cardiovascular complications or events might be averted.

Clinical pearls

- ED is a condition of multifactorial aetiology; as such, the clinician should investigate all factors that could potentially contribute to ED prior to formulating a naturopathic diagnosis and management plan.

- ED can be a clinical manifestation of broader or systemic health issues (e.g. cardiovascular disease). The management of ED therefore needs to take into account managing these broader or systemic health issues in the overall treatment plan.

- Any person presenting with ED of which the aetiology is unknown, the cause is suspected to be serious or managing the condition is out of one's scope of practice, should be referred to an appropriate healthcare professional.

Expert | CONSULT

Clinical Comprehension Questions & Answers are hosted on
**https://expertconsult.inkling.com/store/book/
sarris-clinical-naturopathy-case-files-1**

BIBLIOGRAPHY

Banks E, Joshy G, Abhayaratna WP, et al. Erectile dysfunction severity as a risk marker for cardiovascular disease hospitalisation and all-cause mortality: a prospective cohort study. *PLoS Med.* 2013;10(1):e1001372.

Dickinson HO, Nicolson D, Campbell F, et al. Magnesium supplementation for the management of primary hypertension in adults. *Cochrane Database Sys Rev.* 2006;(3):CD004640.

Gades NM, Nehra A, Jacobson DJ, et al. Association between smoking and erectile dysfunction: a population-based study. *Am J Epidemiol.* 2005;161(4):346-351.

Rees K, Dyakova M, Ward K, et al. Dietary advice for reducing cardiovascular risk. *Cochrane Database Sys Rev.* 2013;(3):CD002128.

Walker AF, Marakis G, Morris AP, et al. Promising hypotensive effect of hawthorn extract: a randomized double-blind pilot study of mild, essential hypertension. *Phytotherapy Res.* 2002;16(1):48-54.

12 Chronic venous insufficiency

Matthew Leach

PRESENTATION

A 68-year-old woman presents with a 15-year history of **bilateral lower limb heaviness, discomfort** and **mild pitting pedal oedema**. The symptoms were relieved 6 years ago following bilateral lower limb venous ligation and stripping; however, they have returned in the past 12 months. The woman is **overweight** (BMI = 28.7 kg/m²), **prehypertensive** (125/85 mmHg), a non-drinker and non-smoker, and has a history of **anxiety** and **chronic constipation**. Her diet is low in dietary fibre, fruit and vegetables, and high in refined carbohydrates. Underlying cardiovascular, lymphatic and renal disease have been excluded.

Diagnostic considerations

Chronic venous insufficiency (CVI) is believed to originate from an episode of macrovascular injury, which may be attributed to lower limb surgery, trauma, deep vein thrombosis (DVT) or pregnancy. This insult to the venous system can lead to valvular incompetence, venous reflux (or retrograde blood flow), ambulatory venous hypertension, venous wall dilation and a subsequent rise in capillary filtration. As well as contributing to the formation of interstitial oedema, increased capillary filtration may also lead to localised hypoxia, malnutrition and eventual tissue destruction. The extravasation of fibrinogen and the consequent formation of pericapillary cuffs, and the intraluminal trapping of leucocytes and subsequent release of toxic metabolites, proteolytic enzymes and tissue necrosis factor alpha (TNF-α), are some of the mechanisms linking elevated capillary filtration pressure to changes in tissue perfusion and local architecture. The extravasation of fibrinogen and leucocyte products into pericapillary tissue may also mediate inflammation, suggesting that CVI may be a disease of chronic inflammation.

SYMPTOMS THAT MAY BE ASSOCIATED WITH OR AGGRAVATE CHRONIC VENOUS INSUFFICIENCY

- Cellulitis
- Congestive heart failure
- DVT
- Hepatic disease
- Hypothyroidism
- Idiopathic oedema
- Lymphoedema
- Renal disease
- Intermittent claudication

Treatment protocol

- The management of CVI primarily focuses on improving venous haemo-dynamics (using venotonic agents or external mechanical force) and/or venous integrity (using agents with antioxidant, anti-inflammatory, antienzymatic and/or antioedema activity).

- *Aesculus hippocastanum* (specifically horse chestnut seed extract standardised to 50–150 mg aescin daily) was reported in a Cochrane review as being more effective than placebo, and as effective as other venotonic agents, at reducing leg pain, oedema, pruritus, leg volume and ankle and calf circumference in patients with mild to moderate CVI, within 20 days to 16 weeks.

- French maritime pine bark extract (pycnogenol) was shown in several randomised controlled trials (RCTs) to be more effective than placebo or compression stockings at reducing leg heaviness and subcutaneous oedema at 8 weeks.

- Standardised red vine leaf extract (from the *Vitis vinifera* Linnaeus vine) has been found to be more effective than placebo at reducing calf circumference, lower limb volume and/or discomfort at 6–12 weeks, according to findings from several RCTs.

- *Ruscus aculeatus* extract was shown in one RCT to be more effective than placebo at reducing leg volume, ankle and leg girth, and leg heaviness, fatigue and tension at 12 weeks. *Centella asiatica* extract has been shown in a systematic review of multiple RCTs to be more effective than placebo at reducing leg heaviness, pain and oedema in 4–8 weeks.

- Mixed bioflavonoids exhibit antioxidant and anti-inflammatory activity in vitro, which may assist in attenuating the progression of venous insufficiency, although this is based on theoretical evidentiary support only.

- Lower limb elevation (to 30 cm above heart level) is likely to offer patients some relief from the symptoms of CVI, although clinical evidence supporting this approach is currently lacking.

- A calf muscle strength exercise program (when used in conjunction with compression hosiery) was shown in one small RCT to improve venous ejection fraction, but not venous reflux, venous severity scores or quality of life, when compared with control.

PRESCRIPTION

Herbal formula (100 mL)

Ruscus aculeatus 1 : 2	35 mL
Centella asiatica 1 : 1	30 mL
Aesculus hippocastanum 1 : 2	25 mL
Zingiber officinale 1 : 2	10 mL

Dose: 7 mL 2 × daily (before meals)

Nutritional prescription

Mixed bioflavonoids (including 500 mg rutin, 500 mg hesperidin and 500 mg quercetin) 2 × daily

Lifestyle prescription

Leg elevation; avoiding prolonged standing; calf muscle strength exercises

Expected outcomes and follow-up protocols

For the 68-year-old woman presenting with CVI, it is unlikely that this chronic condition will ever be cured. The naturopathic treatment approach may, however, prevent further progression of the disease by attenuating the pathogenesis of CVI and, in turn, prevent the development of more serious pathologies, including varicose veins and venous leg ulceration. If the patient adheres to the naturopathic treatment plan (i.e. herbal and nutritional prescription, and lifestyle advice) a clinically significant reduction in CVI manifestations (such as leg heaviness, discomfort and oedema) should be evident within 3 or 4 weeks. If no clinical improvement is observed within this time period, one of the extracts in the herbal prescription should be substituted with *Vaccinium myrtillus*, standarised French maritime pine bark extract, standarised red vine leaf extract or grapeseed extract. Alternatively, the herbal formulation may be replaced with high-dose, enteric-coated horse chestnut seed extract (standardised to 150 mg aescin daily). If the patient continues to be unresponsive to naturopathic treatment after 12 weeks, she should be referred to a vascular surgeon for review.

Clinical pearls

- CVI is a chronic and often disabling disorder of the lower limbs. Effective management of CVI is critical to mitigating the risk of developing varicose veins and/or chronic venous leg ulceration.

- CVI treatment should focus primarily on addressing and resolving the underlying cause and pathological processes of the condition. Naturopathic management of CVI should therefore give preference to agents with venotonic, anti-inflammatory, antioxidant, antienzymatic and antioedema activity and, more importantly, agents with demonstrable clinical efficacy in patients with CVI.

- Any person presenting with signs of CVI of which the aetiology is unknown, arterial insufficiency is suspected or if managing the condition is out of one's scope of practice, should be referred to an appropriate healthcare professional for management and/or further assessment.

Expert|CONSULT

Clinical Comprehension Questions & Answers are hosted on
**https://expertconsult.inkling.com/store/book/
sarris-clinical-naturopathy-case-files-1**

BIBLIOGRAPHY

Chong NJ, Aziz Z. A systematic review of the efficacy of *Centella asiatica* for improvement of the signs and symptoms of chronic venous insufficiency. *Evid Based Complement Alternat Med.* 2013;2013(2013):Art. ID., 627182.

Padberg FT, Johnston MV, Sisto SA. Structured exercise improves calf muscle pump function in chronic venous insufficiency: a randomized trial. *J Vasc Surg.* 2004;39(1):79-87.

Pappas PJ, Lal BK, Cerveira JJ, et al. Causes of severe chronic venous insufficiency. *Semin Vasc Surg.* 2005;18:30-35.

Pittler MH, Ernst E. Horse chestnut seed extract for chronic venous insufficiency. *Cochrane Database Syst Rev.* 2012;(11):Art. No.: CD003230.

Rabe E, Stucker M, Esperester A, et al. Efficacy and tolerability of a red-vine-leaf extract in patients suffering from chronic venous insufficiency – results of a double-blind placebo-controlled study. *Eur J Vasc Surg.* 2011;41(4):540-547.

Vanscheidt W, Jost V, Wolna P, et al. Efficacy and safety of a butcher's broom preparation (*Ruscus aculeatus* L. extract) compared to placebo in patients suffering from chronic venous insufficiency. *Arzneimittelforschung.* 2002;52(4):243-250.

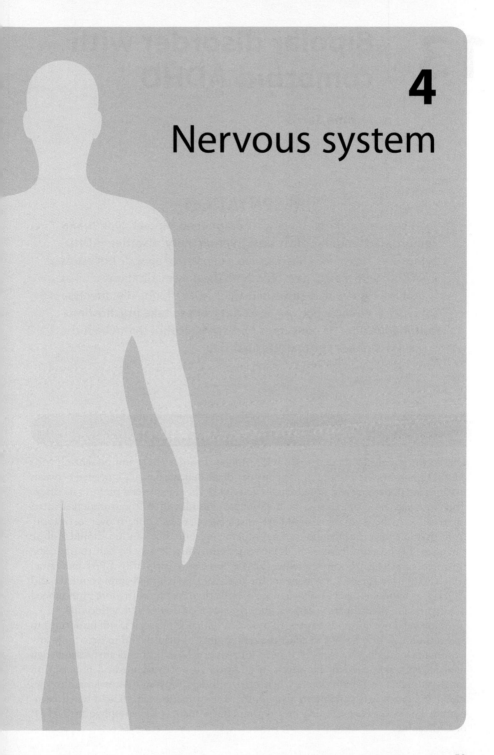

4

Nervous system

Bipolar disorder with comorbid ADHD

Jerome Sarris

PRESENTATION

A 24-year-old male presents with **diagnosed bipolar type II and comorbid attention deficit and hyperactivity disorder (ADHD) symptoms**. He recently has resolved a depressive episode but wants assistance with maintaining his mood. The only medication he takes is lithium. He has had suspected mild ADHD (primarily attention subtype) since childhood but **does not want to take psychostimulant medication**. He **consumes excessive alcohol** throughout the week and **smokes 10 cigarettes per day**.

Diagnostic considerations

Due to the patient being diagnosed with bipolar disorder (BD) and presenting with ADHD symptoms, it is important to consider that a delicate balance is needed between modulating dopamine and noradrenalin activity in the dorsolateral prefrontal cortex. This area may be overactivated in hypomanic episodes in BD and underactivated in ADHD. As he is taking a mood stabiliser, there is less concern over 'activation' from thymoleptic treatments into a hypomanic episode, but caution should still be extended. In the above case, as he is currently euthymic, it may be best to prescribe treatments such as N-acetylcysteine (NAC), omega-3 (primarily EPA) and zinc, which may have longer term benefits for both BD (and mood improvement) and ADHD, as opposed to prescribing a more specific thymoleptic with more pronounced antidepressant effects such as *Hypericum perforatum* or S-adenosylmethionine.

While he is not currently depressed or in a hypomanic phase, it is still important to take a thorough case history to chart the temporality of his BD and to determine any hypomanic or depressive triggers. If symptoms of psychosis or mania are present, then medical referral is needed. However, in addition to potential medical prescription for hypo/mania (e.g. high potency benzodiazepines, antipsychotics or an additional mood stabiliser) it is possible to also adjunctively prescribe amino acid-based compounds known to have calming or sedating effects such as L-tryptophan or 5-HTP, or L-theanine.

Regarding the presence of ADHD symptoms, it is important to first confirm a diagnosis of ADHD (the symptoms need to be significant enough and to have started in childhood) and to rule out any other underlying primary psychiatric or medical causes. It is also helpful to take a complete history to determine a possible relationship between diet, food allergies, etc. (including food colourings or additives) and the ADHD symptoms.

IMPORTANT DIAGNOSTIC/CLINICAL CONSIDERATIONS

- When patients present with depression, be aware that this may be a depressive phase of BD
- If involved in managing a patient with bipolar hypo/mania, be aware that a depressive phase may occur after the 'high' has resolved
- Treatment of depression is vital to reduce risk of suicide and improve quality of life for the patient
- ADHD may occur comorbidly with BD; in such cases it is a delicate balance between stimulating and sedating/regulating certain neuro-chemical pathways

Treatment protocol

- To assist in the maintenance of mood, adjunctive use of omega-3 and zinc may be prescribed alongside his mood stabiliser lithium. These have demonstrated a beneficial effect on depressive, but not manic, symptoms.

- While omega-3 has had mixed evidence for use in ADHD, it is still vital to be prescribed in a deficient diet, and evidence supports its adjunctive use with pharmacotherapy, providing an anti-inflammatory action with a modulatory effect on several neurotransmitter systems.

- Zinc is critical for neurological and endocrinological function and has an important role in many enzymatic reactions. Zinc prescription also supports immune function and modulates the inflammatory cascade.

- Increased oxidative stress and inflammation may also play a role in BD and ADHD. NAC is known to replenish brain levels of glutathione, the brain's major free-radical scavenger. This may be beneficial in both BD and ADHD.

- To assist in mood maintenance and improve overall general health, regular exercise and mind–body practices are advised. This will provide a healthy preventative framework for patients diagnosed with either BD or ADHD.

- Ongoing psychoeducation about the importance of lifestyle and stress management, together with support groups and other psychosocial interventions, may enhance his treatment adherence and aid in the recognition and response to early warning signs of relapse.

- Smoking cigarettes is a potential risk factor for depression via aberration of the dopaminergic system and increased inflammation and oxidative stress. Reduction or elimination of smoking is a vital lifestyle recommendation.

- Reducing his alcohol consumption is also important because there is a two-way relationship between alcohol consumption and depressed mood (although this is not conclusive). A brief education intervention (providing safe drinking guidance), potentially via online education or appropriate referral, may also be of benefit.

PRESCRIPTION
Nutritional prescription

NAC: 2.4 g–3 g per day (1200 mg–1500 mg 2 × daily)
Zinc amino acid chelate (or picolinate): 30 mg elemental per day (2 × 15 mg tablets)
Omega-3 containing high EPA (1 g of EPA per day)

Lifestyle prescription

Regular exercise and time in nature
Good sleep hygiene
Reduction/elimination of nicotine and alcohol
Wholefood (non-processed) diet
Mindfulness training

Expected outcomes and follow-up protocols

The treatment of BD may be an ongoing process, and naturopathic clinicians should be aware of the need for an integrative approach that may combine pharmacotherapy (especially in BD type I) and psychological intervention, in addition to lifestyle modification and judicious nutraceutical prescription. If the patient has a hypomanic episode, stabilisation of mood must be firstly achieved via medical intervention. When approaching an acutely manic patient the principal treatment goals are patient safety and rapid stabilisation; this frequently requires psychiatric hospitalisation. Clinical management decisions regarding the use of adjunctive nutraceuticals should always be accompanied by careful monitoring for warning signs of recurring hypomanic, depressive or psychotic episodes and treatment-emergent adverse effects, or drug interactions. Lithium has a narrow therapeutic range and may have some deleterious effects on the endocrine and urinary systems. Due to this, lithium blood levels, interaction with other pharmacotherapies (including nutraceuticals) and effects on general health needs to be monitored.

While it is ill-advised to recommend he stop taking his lithium without medical approval, adjunctive use of the above prescription may potentially permit lower effective doses of mood stabilisers, reduced incidence of adverse effects and improved medication compliance over the long term. Ongoing psychoeducation or psychosocial interventions may enhance treatment adherence and help bipolar patients recognise and respond to early warning signs of relapse.

In terms of treating his ADHD symptoms, while psychostimulants remain the frontline evidence-based approach (and no nutraceuticals have revealed consistent equivalent effects), his ADHD symptoms are mild and manageable, thus this approach may not be needed. His attention issues may improve via the above prescription, in addition to lifestyle modification and mindfulness/attention training. People with bipolar disorder II can live productive and happy lives; however, ongoing mood management may be needed. Any integrative treatment approach needs to be adjusted according to hypomania/depression/euthymia phases, with a view to tailoring treatment to individual preference, tolerability and financial considerations.

Clinical pearls

- Available conventional pharmacological treatments for the depressive phase of BD have limited efficacy and some potential safety issues, in addition to common noncompliance. Therefore an integrated approach is advised.

- Evidence suggests that NAC, omega-3 fatty acids and zinc may have potential adjunctive use in improving mood in people with depression.

- Zinc supplementation may be helpful when hyperactivity and impulsive behaviour do not respond to stimulants alone.

- Regular exercise, relaxation training, yoga or other mind–body practices and psychoeducation may help reduce relapse risk in some cases of BD.

Expert | CONSULT

Clinical Comprehension Questions & Answers are hosted on
**https://expertconsult.inkling.com/store/book/
sarris-clinical-naturopathy-case-files-1**

BIBLIOGRAPHY

Berk M, Malhi GS, Gray LJ, et al. The promise of N-acetylcysteine in neuropsychiatry. *Trends Pharmacol Sci.* 2013;34(3):167-177.

Murray G, Suto M, Hole R, et al. Self-management strategies used by 'high functioning' individuals with bipolar disorder: from research to clinical practice. *Clin Psychol Psychother.* 2010;EPub.

Sarris J, Kean J, Schweitzer I, et al. Complementary medicines (herbal and nutritional products) in the treatment of attention deficit hyperactivity disorder (ADHD): a systematic review of the evidence. *Complement Ther Med.* 2011;19(4):216-227.

Sarris J, Lake J, Hoenders R. Bipolar disorder and complementary medicine: current evidence, safety issues, and clinical considerations. *J Altern Complement Med.* 2011;17(10):881-890.

Sarris J, Mischoulon D, Schweitzer I. Adjunctive nutraceuticals with standard pharmacotherapies in bipolar disorder: a systematic review of clinical trials. *Bipolar Disord.* 2011;13(5-6):454-465.

14 Chronic anxiety with comorbid insomnia

Jerome Sarris

PRESENTATION

A 38-year-old female presents with **chronic anxiety** and worsening **insomnia**. She says she has felt tense and anxious over the past 2 years and constantly worries. Over the past month she has had **digestive issues** (nausea and cramping worsened by stress) and regular **heart palpitations**. Sleep has been persistently worse (5–6 hours of broken sleep and wakes unrefreshed). Due to a **busy life** and high work demands she **eats spasmodically** and consumes a lot of **fast food** and **caffeine**.

Diagnostic considerations

In the above case, there is the likelihood that the patient is suffering from generalised anxiety disorder. This is manifesting as chronic worry, digestive issues, heart palpitations and physical and psychological tension, in addition to it affecting her sleep. Aside from a thorough assessment of triggering/worsening factors, timeline and general symptoms, it is important to refer for a thyroid test to rule out hyperthyroidism.

The initial goal is to reduce the patient's anxiety as soon as possible. This should be able to be achieved via a combination of an anxiolytic herbal medicine prescription and lifestyle changes. Long term, while it may be difficult to alleviate work pressures (unless changing jobs), it is possible via meditative or mindfulness practice and psychological techniques such as cognitive behaviour therapy to modify the stress response to this. In respect to sleep, insomnia is common in anxiety sufferers, and treating this is of primary importance as poor sleep may in turn deleteriously affect neuroendocrine balance and subsequently exacerbate the anxiety. Therefore treating her anxiety should improve sleep and, in turn, better sleep should lessen anxiety. Better quality sleep should allow for a reduction in caffeine consumption, which may also reduce anxiety symptoms.

IMPORTANT DIAGNOSTIC/CLINICAL CONSIDERATIONS
- Screen for anxiety disorders
- Consider thyroid dysfunction
- Be aware of the potential for anxiety to develop into depression later
- Monitor for alcohol or stimulant misuse
- Lifestyle modification and psychological techniques are essential

Treatment protocol

- The herbal prescription is designed to primarily exert anxiolytic, adaptogenic and spasmolytic activity. *Piper methysticum* is used as the premier anxiety-reducing herbal medicine in the formula. This can be used twice a day or as needed, although with any long-term use occasional liver function tests are advised. *Piper methysticum* should not be taken in concert with alcohol or benzodiazepines. *Passiflora incarnata* and *Scutellaria lateriflora* will also augment this effect. *Withania somnifera* provides a non-stimulating adaptogenic tonic and anxiolytic action. Magnesium may be of benefit as an adjunctive anxiolytic and spasmolytic, as her diet is likely to be low in this mineral. This can be prescribed away from meals and in combination with calcium if the diet is also low in this mineral.

- While dietary programs designed to assist in reducing anxiety have to date not been rigorously evaluated, dietary improvement is advised in this case. A basic balanced diet with foods rich in individual nutrients such as folate, omega-3, tryptophan, zinc, magnesium and B and C vitamins can be recommended. These foods include whole grains, lean meat, deep-sea fish, green leafy vegetables, coloured berries and nuts (walnuts, almonds). A low glycaemic index diet may be beneficial in stabilising blood sugar levels, which may in turn reduce the 'fight or flight' response of low blood sugar levels.

- General lifestyle advice should focus on encouraging a balance between meaningful work, judicious exercise and adequate rest and sleep. Physical activity is anecdotally regarded as having a positive effect on reducing stress and anxiety, with people often participating in activities such as walking, swimming, cycling, yoga or gym training in order to improve their wellbeing. Graded exercise programs that may be appropriate for reducing anxiety may involve either aerobic or anabolic exercise for a minimum of 20 minutes three to five times a week.

- In respect to addressing sleep issues, this should be improved as her anxiety resolves. However, as part of an integrative approach, the use of hypnotic, anxiolytic and adaptogenic actions in the formula should help restore sleep (all herbal medicines listed in the prescription have a potential mildly sedating/hypnotic effect if taken in the evening). This, in combination with good sleep hygiene techniques, should facilitate sleep. The use of L-tryptophan (or 5-HTP) or melatonin may also be potential options for the evening (these may, however, have restricted use in some jurisdictions).

- To further address her sleep issues, sleep hygiene techniques are advised. The key techniques revealed by sleep researchers focuses primarily on limiting exposure to the bed (sleep restriction). This could mean having only a limited time to sleep and getting up at a set time in the morning regardless of quality or quantity of sleep. The other mainstay is to reduce exposure to light prior to sleep and to increase exposure to morning sunlight upon waking. It is also best to avoid excessive daytime naps as this may disturb the circadian rhythm. Additional sleep hygiene advice includes stimulus control—that is, avoidance of stimulating activity and stimulants close to sleep such as smoking, caffeine and external stimuli (stimulating TV or books).

- Positive social interaction and pleasurable hobbies are also advised. Behavioural therapy techniques have shown beneficial effects on reducing anxiety by training the person to reduce or better manage stressful situations, and to increase pleasurable activities. These may enhance self-esteem and self-mastery, and increase physical and mental wellbeing.

- Removal of caffeine is a vital component to reduce anxiety and improve sleep. Caffeine causes arousal, hypervigilance and possible anxiogenesis in certain individuals via stimulation of beta-adrenergic receptors and up-regulation of nor/adrenalin and dopamine, while adenosine receptor antagonism interferes with sleep.

- Patients may also be advised to keep a worry or sleep diary to record their worries and sleep pattern.

Expected outcomes and follow-up protocols

In the above case the patient's anxiety is expected to reduce shortly after beginning *Piper methysticum* and the herbal formula, which should have a quick onset of activity. The prognosis is better if the course of anxiety is not complicated by comorbid mental disorders or substance abuse, or if there is a history of chronic persistent anxiety. An integrative approach involving psychological, dietary/nutraceutical, lifestyle and herbal interventions should offer a sustained benefit if compliance is maintained. If after 2 weeks minimal benefit occurs, the herbal prescription can be modified to include other potential anxiolytics such as *Melissa officinalis, Bacopa monnieri, Magnolia* spp. or *Ginkgo biloba*. Additional psychological interventions may also be of assistance—that is, behavioural or social-based models to examine and aid in managing external triggers of the anxiety.

PRESCRIPTION
Herbal formula (100 mL)

Withania somnifera 1:1	40 mL
Passiflora incarnata 1:2	25 mL
Scutellaria lateriflora 1:2	20 mL
Matricaria recutita 1:2	15 mL

Dose: 7.5 mL 2 × daily

Piper methysticum (aqueous extract containing 60 mg kavalactones)
2 tablets 2 × daily

Nutritional prescription

Magnesium amino acid chelate: (100 mg elemental) 2 tablets 2 × daily

Lifestyle prescription

Graded exercise
Dietary modification
Good sleep hygiene
Reduced caffeine

The patient's insomnia is expected to be ameliorated within a week or two. As is the case with anxiety, chronic insomniacs have a poorer prognosis if it is complicated by comorbid mental disorders or substance abuse. If after 2 weeks minimal benefit has occurred, the herbal prescription can be modified to include a specific 'sleep formula' with hypnotics such as *Valeriana* spp., *Ziziphus jujuba*, *Humulus lupulus* or *Eschscholzia californica*. The use of melatonin or L-tryptophan (or 5-HTP) may also be used if the patient is non-responsive to the initial prescription. 'Judicious' use of pharmaceutical hypnotics may also be considered if anxiety, panic or poor sleep continues in order to minimise suffering, although consideration of potential addiction and withdrawal effects need to be monitored.

Clinical pearls

- Anxiety disorders are commonly comorbid with many psychiatric disorders.

- Screen for substance, stimulant and alcohol misuse.

- Realise the potential for chronic anxiety to lead on to a depressive episode.

- Reduce anxiety initially via an appropriate prescription, and integrate lifestyle modifications over time.

Expert | **CONSULT**

Clinical Comprehension Questions & Answers are hosted on
**https://expertconsult.inkling.com/store/book/
sarris-clinical-naturopathy-case-files-1**

BIBLIOGRAPHY

Huh J, Goebert D, Takeshita J, et al. Treatment of generalized anxiety disorder: a comprehensive review of the literature for psychopharmacologic alternatives to newer antidepressants and benzodiazepines. *Prim Care Companion CNS Disord.* 2011;13:2.

Sarris J, Byrne GJ. A systematic review of insomnia and complementary medicine. *Sleep Med Rev.* 2011;15(2):99-106.

Sarris J, LaPorte E, Schweitzer I. Kava: a comprehensive review of efficacy, safety, and psychopharmacology. *Aust N Z J Psychiatry.* 2011;45(1):27-35.

Sarris J, Moylan S, Camfield DA, et al. Complementary medicine, exercise, meditation, diet, and lifestyle modification for anxiety disorders: a review of current evidence. *Evid Based Complement Alternat Med.* 2012;2012:809653.

Sarris J, McIntyre E, Camfield DA. Plant-based medicines for anxiety disorders, part 2: a review of clinical studies with supporting preclinical evidence. *CNS Drugs.* 2013;27(4):301-319.

15 Clinical depression

Jerome Sarris

PRESENTATION

A 42-year-old female presents with a primary complaint of **persistent low mood for the past 3 months**, in addition to feeling physically **wound up** and **anxious**. No signs of current or previous mania/hypomania are noted. She mentions that recently **her memory and mental function has been diminishing**. She says that she isn't positive about life and has very negative self-talk. Her **diet is poor**, lacking in leafy vegetables, fruits and whole grains. The patient reports **very low levels of physical activity**. Tests reveal that thyroid function is normal, as is salivary cortisol.

Diagnostic considerations

Treatment of the above case should involve aiming to improve mood, in addition to ameliorating anxiety. Unipolar depression is evident here, with the anxiety presenting comorbidly as a potential co-occurring anxiety disorder (e.g. generalised anxiety disorder), or as anxious symptomatology as a manifestation of the clinical depression. In this case, a treatment approach that provides mood elevation needs to be modified to not overstimulate her. Interventions that modulate the serotonergic and GABAergic pathways may therefore be indicated. In cases presenting with fatigue, apathy and somnolence with no comorbid anxiety, an approach targeting noradrenergic and dopaminergic pathways may be indicated.

Her poor memory may also be a reflection of cognitive impairment from depression; however, if it is still occurring after amelioration of depression or if co-occurring with headaches, medical referral is advised. When treating depression it is critical to screen for suicidality and refer if appropriate. It is also important to screen for other co-occurring psychiatric disorders and to refer for tests if warranted to rule out an underlying biological pathology (e.g. brain tumour). Alcohol and substance misuse is common with depression, and this can also be a causative factor.

IMPORTANT DIAGNOSTIC/CLINICAL CONSIDERATIONS
- Hypothyroidism or hyperthyroidism
- Bipolarity and suicidal ideation
- Rule out any causes of depression from medication or medical conditions
- Monitor the course of the illness for changes in mood, sleep, anxiety levels and substance or alcohol misuse
- Antidepressant medication may be needed if depressive episodes worsen and persist

Treatment protocol

- The primary approach is to provide an antidepressant action to treat the depression. In the above case, a dysregulation of serotonin pathways may be responsible for the low mood and anxiety, therefore the prescription of *Hypericum perforatum* and S-adenosylmethionine (SAMe) is of potential benefit. *Rhodiola rosea* can also be considered; however, this patient needs to be monitored for overstimulation.

- To address comorbid anxiety *Passiflora incarnata* is added, in addition to magnesium for reducing muscular tension and for neurochemical function (also addresses any dietary deficiency). It is intended that the *Passiflora* may mitigate any hyperstimulatory effects from the *Rhodiola*.

- *Ginkgo biloba* may provide a beneficial nootropic effect, in addition to supplementary anxiolytic activity.

- General lifestyle advice should focus on encouraging a balance between meaningful work, adequate rest/sleep, judicious exercise, hobbies and pleasurable social interaction.

- Cognitive behaviour therapy (CBT) techniques can be used (or referral for) promoting positive and balanced cognition. This addresses an important psychological component of depression. This may take the form of mindfulness-based CBT. This can be taught by a trained clinician or referred out (online e-therapy may also be an option).

- Dietary advice is crucial, especially the addition of sufficient protein, which provides the nutrient building blocks for neurochemicals and enzymes involved in mood maintenance. Judicious use or avoidance of caffeine may also be appropriate as caffeine may aggravate anxiety.

- Omega-3 fatty acids are advised via an increase of deep-sea oily fish (at least two 100 g portions per week) and polyunsaturated-rich seeds from the diet or via supplementation if needed (high EPA formulations advised).

PRESCRIPTION

Herbal formula (100 mL)

Hypericum perforatum 1:2	25 mL
Rhodiola rosea 2:1	25 mL
Passiflora incarnata 1:2	25 mL
Ginkgo biloba 2:1	25 mL
Dose: 5 mL 3 × daily	

Nutritional prescription

SAMe: 2 tablets 2 × daily (800 mg)
Magnesium amino acid chelate: 2 tablets (80 mg elemental) 2 × daily

Lifestyle prescription

Moderate balanced exercise
Good sleep hygiene
Mindfulness meditation
Dietary improvement

Expected outcomes and follow-up protocols

It is vital when treating depression to follow up with the patient soon after beginning a new prescription (to monitor for changes in mood and to provide additional psychological support). In the above case, reduction of depression and a return towards euthymia is expected within a month of commencing treatment (although most people will show some initial signs of improvement early if treatment is likely to be effective). Many people will have some of their depression alleviated simply by taking the step to seek treatment, making lifestyle adjustments, and from the interpersonal therapeutic relationship with the practitioner. If the depressive episode persists beyond 4–6 weeks and suicidality is still absent, a change of prescription is required. Additional interventions such as 5-HTP, zinc or EPA (omega-3), or electroacupuncture, may be potentially helpful. Addressing the diet via increased whole foods and prebiotic and probiotic foods may be beneficial for bowel health and the microbiome composition.

If the condition worsens then medical referral is advised, with a prescription of antidepressants being potentially warranted. In the case of antidepressant medication being commenced, the naturopathic treatment protocol can be in essence maintained; however, *Hypericum perforatum* should be discontinued, and use of other serotonergic agents such as 5-HTP should be monitored closely. The prescription can be adjusted to address several potential commonly occurring side effects from antidepressants such as nausea, insomnia and sexual dysfunction. The patient can also be assessed for lower folate metabolism in homozygous carriers of the MTHR C677T and A1298C SNPs (with folinic acid or methylfolate being prescribed).

Depressive episodes are often diagnostically unstable, therefore the patient should be monitored carefully to modulate the prescription according to any changes in symptoms. Changes that may occur include the emergence of hypo/mania, anxiety, insomnia or alterations in appetite, energy or cognition. After the depressive symptoms remit, treatment can be continued for 3–6 months to potentially enhance the chance of sustained remission.

Clinical pearls

- While diagnosing depression, rule out other medical diagnoses such as hypothyroidism, anaemia or infectious diseases that could mimic some signs of depression.

- Always investigate the use of alcohol and drugs when evaluating for mood disorders.

- The addition of any new medication should be investigated to ensure it is not contributing to the patient's symptoms.

- Always screen for suicidal ideation and symptoms of bipolarity in patients with low mood.

Expert | CONSULT

Clinical Comprehension Questions & Answers are hosted on
https://expertconsult.inkling.com/store/book/
sarris-clinical-naturopathy-case-files-1

BIBLIOGRAPHY

Quirk S. The association between diet quality, dietary patterns and depression in adults: a systematic review. *BMC Psychiatry*. 2014;13:175.

Sarris J. 'Clinical depression: an evidence-based integrative complementary medicine treatment model'. *Altern Ther Health Med*. 2011;17(4):26-37.

Sarris J, Kavanagh DJ, Byrne G. 'Adjuvant use of nutritional and herbal medicines with antidepressants, mood stabilizers and benzodiazepines'. *J Psychiatr Res*. 2010;44(1):32-41.

Sarris J, Panossian A, Schweitzer I, et al. 'Herbal medicine for depression, anxiety and insomnia: a review of psychopharmacology and clinical evidence'. *Eur Neuropsychopharmacol*. 2011;21(12):841-860.

Sarris J, O'Neil A, Coulson CE, et al. 'Lifestyle medicine for depression'. *BMC Psychiatry*. 2013;10(14):107.

16 | Migraine (nervous)

Phil Cottingham

PRESENTATION

A 68-year-old female presents with **migraines** that manifest on the vertex or behind either eye. However, several other **comorbidities** are critical to understanding the case. She is **overweight** and has been for some time. She suffers from **asthma** and **sinusitis** and **low thyroid** (she talks softly and appears slightly retiring).

Diagnostic considerations

The key diagnostic consideration is differentiating between headache and migraine. Headache is defined as pain in the cranial region, an isolated benign occurrence or manifestation of a variety of disorders, whereas migraine is defined as a disabling, primary headache that is characterised by unilateral pulsating pain. Headache is more generalised pain; migraine is unilateral and generally produces several concomitant symptoms. Although a detailed definition of headache disorders is evolving (and remains somewhat controversial) the basics of differentiation between headache and migraine remain reasonably constant.

Aura alone is not a defining factor in this differential diagnosis, as migraine is also defined as being with or without aura (premonition of the pain and other symptoms).

Once a definition of migraine has been established, there is a need to check for migraine risk and trigger factors. Weight is a common comorbidity with migraine, as is bipolar disorder. The thyroid should be tested regularly (thyroid-stimulating hormone, total thyroid and free T3/T4 tests). Clinical manifestations of low thyroid (such as weight gain, constipation, dry skin, fatigue and loss of appetite) need to be monitored regularly. Asthma and sinusitis should be monitored, especially for secondary infection. Mood monitoring for bipolar disorder could be useful, particularly if it is occurring in relation to migraine.

MEDICAL CONDITIONS THAT MAY MIMIC OR AGGRAVATE MIGRAINES AND HEADACHE SYMPTOMS

- Acute respiratory infection
- Cerebral venous thrombosis
- Subarachnoid or intracranial haemorrhage
- Meningitis or encephalitis
- Glaucoma
- Benign intracranial hypertension
- Spinal disorders such as cervical spondylosis
- Sinusitis
- Trauma to the head or neck/shoulder region
- Depression or psychogenic disorders
- Diabetes
- Drug-induced headache
- Anaemia
- Thyroid disorder
- Urinary tract infection

Treatment protocol

- Nutritional counselling is central to the treatment protocol. Addressing trigger foods (low inflammatory) is the initial focus, but also addressing deficiencies, adding nutrient-positive foods (e.g. vegetables, nuts and seeds, legumes, low-glycaemic fruits and whole grains in moderation), gradual weight loss and maintenance of blood sugar levels and hydration are all important.

- To address migraine prophylaxis *Tanacetum parthenium* or *Petasites hybridus* can be prescribed, while *Fucus vesiculosus* is prescribed for thyroid function.

- *Zingiber officinale* is prescribed for its anti-inflammatory and antiemetic effects, and to dampen inflammatory immune responses in the digestive tract (which are also addressed using *Hydrastis canadensis*).

- Magnesium is prescribed to help relax smooth muscle tissue.

- The patient is counselled to exercise more, especially after dinner, which will allow for better digestion and assist weight loss.

- Regular massage treatments are advised to increase blood flow and reduce tension (especially in the cervical region). A referral for craniosacral therapy is also advised, especially to create greater mobility between cranial bones, the occipital bone and cervical spine, and to assist with blood flow from the head (through venous sinuses).

PRESCRIPTION
Herbal formula (100 mL)

Tanacetum parthenium 1:5	30 mL
Fucus vesiculosus 1:1	30 mL
Hydrastis canadensis 1:3	25 mL
Zingiber officinale 1:2	15 mL
Dose: 5 mL 3 × daily	

Nutritional prescription

Magnesium citrate: 300 mg (84 mg approx. elemental magnesium) 2 × daily

Lifestyle prescription

Moderate balanced exercise
Dietary improvement
Physical/mobility therapy

Expected outcomes and follow-up protocols

Gradual improvement is expected. In such complex cases, several factors will affect the rate of improvement, and it is important to monitor each symptom carefully. Initially there should be a change in intensity of the migraine, but frequency may also improve over the next few months.

Weight loss would be very gradual and may fluctuate due to the patient's age and the mental health effects of the condition (especially if the patient is taking a mood stabiliser or antipsychotic medication for management of bipolar disorder). Her weight should be monitored sensitively so as not to create distress. Blood sugar should be monitored in the clinic at each visit and changes noted; this may influence alterations in treatment and herbal prescription. The effects of the craniosacral treatment need to be carefully assessed. This can be done with regular communication (written and oral) with the therapist, who can monitor the effects of the massage treatment.

This case will require long-term management, and her bipolar disorder also needs to be monitored and managed with collaborative psychiatric care. The patient's age and lifestyle will exert a considerable influence on the outcomes, but the integrated nature of the approach will ensure improvements, albeit gradual.

Clinical pearls

- When assessing a patient with headache it is important to differentiate between the main types and the subtypes.

- Always investigate triggers and remember that, while there are immediate triggers (coffee, chocolate, etc.), dietary considerations should also investigate foods that are frequently consumed (even if not a known migraine or headache trigger). Consider eliminating certain foods and conducting a challenge test (with caution to ensure there is not an overreaction to those foods).

- Ask the patient to get a test for the presence of *Helicobacter pylori*, as this has been shown in recent research to be present in 40% of migraine sufferers, and consider herbal treatment for this pathogen if the test is positive.

Expert | CONSULT

Clinical Comprehension Questions & Answers are hosted on **https://expertconsult.inkling.com/store/book/ sarris-clinical-naturopathy-case-files-1**

BIBLIOGRAPHY

Bigal M, Lipton R. Modifiable risk factors for migraine progression. *Headache: J Head Face Pain.* 2006;46(9):1334-1343.

Cottingham P. Headache and migraine. In: Sarris J, Wardle J, eds. *Clinical Naturopathy: an Evidence-Based Guide to Practice.* 2nd ed. Chatswood. NSW: Churchill Livingstone; 2014.

Lipton R, Göbel H, Einhäupl K, et al. Petasites hybridus root (butterbur) is an effective preventive treatment for migraine. *Neurology.* 2004;63(12):2240-2244.

Maizels M, Blumenfeld A, Burchette R. Combination of riboflavin, magnesium, and feverfew for migraine prophylaxis: a randomized trial. *Headache: J Head Face Pain.* 2004;44(9):885-890.

Peterlin B, Rosso A, Rapoport A, et al. Obesity and migraine: the effect of age, gender and adipose tissue distribution. *Headache: J Head Face Pain.* 2010;50(1):52-62.

Ageing and cognition

Christina Kure

PRESENTATION

A 68-year-old male presents with **concerns about forgetting daily tasks**. He is semi-retired, working 3 days per week. He reports feeling **stressed and anxious about money and retirement**. He does not have difficulty getting to sleep but **wakes at night** with **worrying thoughts** and **nocturnal urination** and cannot get back to sleep. He **gets tired easily** during the day. He drinks three beers and two glasses of wine 5 nights per week, drinks three or four espressos per day, has an active social life and travels for leisure regularly. Concomitant conditions include **osteoarthritis in the knees, hands and fingers** and **lower back pain**. He has been cleared of Alzheimer's disease (via neuroimaging and neuropsychological testing).

Diagnostic considerations

The primary naturopathic treatment goal should be to enhance cognitive function (attention and memory), reduce stress and improve sleep quality using a combination of herbal, nutritional, dietary and lifestyle interventions. However, other conditions include depression, which is associated with poor memory, poor concentration and reduced ability to adequately undertake daily activities. This needs to be considered as part of the differential diagnosis.

Other conditions including major depressive disorder, cerebrovascular disease, cardiovascular disease and a history of transient ischaemic attacks or stroke also need to be ruled out.

Referral to a medical practitioner may be required for detailed medical appraisal to exclude more severe conditions and possible referral to a clinical psychologist for a detailed cognitive assessment. However, in the above case cognitive decline associated with the natural ageing process is the most likely diagnosis. Fatigue and stress may also be impacting on the poor memory and attention, and the treatment approach therefore needs to also address these concomitant symptoms. Therefore, a secondary treatment goal is to address risk factors that may be attributing to the presenting symptoms (e.g. excessive alcohol intake and inflammation) and comorbid conditions including arthritic and physical pain to improve mobility, associated pain and general quality of life.

IMPORTANT DIAGNOSTIC/CLINICAL CONSIDERATIONS

- Presence of depression or clinical anxiety
- Sleep issues/insomnia
- Fatigue levels
- Comorbid pain
- Cardiovascular risk factors (metabolic syndrome, type 2 diabetes)

Treatment protocol

- The primary treatment goal in the short term is to improve sleep quality, decrease stress and improve energy levels during the day. Begin treatment with nutraceuticals that may enhance cognition.

- *Bacopa monnieri* and *Ginkgo biloba* may improve cognitive function.

- *Passiflora incarnata*, *Humulus lupulus*, *Scutellaria lateriflora* and *Piper methysticum* may improve quality of sleep and reduce anxiety and in turn combat feelings of tiredness.

- Traditionally used as a nervine tonic, *Melissa officinalis* may be beneficial for decreasing the agitation and anxiety, with added cognitive benefits.

- Address nutritional deficiencies with antioxidant compounds such as alpha-lipoic acid and vitamins C, E, D and B. Folic acid will provide additional therapeutic support.

- Recommend a diet that follows the principles of a Mediterranean diet (rich in olive oil, vegetables, legumes, cereals and fruit, nuts and seeds, and low in animal fats and products, one to two serves of fish per week, low consumption of dairy and moderate amounts of wine).

- Increasing polyphenols such as organic berries (blueberries, strawberries) either raw or in a smoothie, tea (green tea, black tea), small amounts of cocoa (dark organic chocolate) and turmeric is recommended.

- Green tea and foods rich in vitamins C, E and B including folate need to be increased.

- Encourage participation in cognitively-stimulating activities such as reading the newspaper and doing crosswords.

- Regular light–moderate exercise (e.g. walking, gardening, aerobic fitness training) should be encouraged to improve cognitive function, lift mood, assist with sleep and strengthen the muscular and vascular systems.

- Address concomitant conditions, particularly arthritis, with glucosamine and chondroitin, alternatives, circulatory stimulants and/or topical analgesics.

PRESCRIPTION
Main herbal formula (100 mL)

Bacopa monnieri 1:2	25 mL
Ginkgo biloba 2:1	25 mL
Melissa officinalis 1:2	20 mL
Panax ginseng 1:2	25 mL
Rosmarinus officinalis 1.2	5 mL
Dose: 5 mL 3 × daily	

Sleep and anxiety herbal formula (50 mL)

Melissa officinalis 1:2	15 mL
Humulus lupulus	15 mL
Scutellaria lateriflora	20 mL
5 mL 1 hour before bedtime	

Nutritional prescription

Glucosamine (750 mg) and chondroitin (225 mg) 2 × daily

Lifestyle prescription

Gradually reduce alcohol intake to one standard drink per day
Moderate physical activity; reduce sitting time
Progressive muscle relaxation or meditation
Green tea: 1–2 cups per day

Expected outcomes and follow-up protocols

By addressing sleep disturbances and stress, expect some improvements in memory during the first 2 weeks. Expect more prominent improvements 4–6 weeks after commencing the herbal formula, and sleep patterns would be expected to improve after 1 week of taking the sleep mix. Regardless, it is important to pursue additional medical assessments if his cognition does not improve, or worsens.

Additionally, body work such as remedial massage, osteopathy or remedial massage is recommended to address back and arthritic pain. Treating the osteoarthritis with glucosamine and chondroitin, circulatory stimulants or anti-inflammatories (e.g. *Zingiber officinale*, *Boswellia serrata*) can also be initiated early on to allow time for the treatments to have the desired effect (at least 1 month). By treating his physical pain (back pain), expect the insomnia and symptoms of anxiety, the attention issues and forgetfulness to potentially improve. If nocturnal urination persists

1 week after not drinking fluids in the evening and reducing alcohol and caffeine intake, consider reevaluating urinary system function, and treat any imbalances with appropriate urinary herbs.

Financial planning and counselling on end-of-life issues may be beneficial to help ease stress and anxieties. The treatment protocol needs to be reassessed after 2 weeks if no improvements are seen in sleep, energy levels during the day or stress; prescribe hypnotics (sleep) or adaptogenics and 'nervines' such as *Piper methysticum*, *Avena sativa* or *Withania somnifera*. Additionally, reassess the treatment protocol after 2 months if deterioration is seen in any aspect of cognitive function, stress levels or mood. A treatment that the patient responds well to should be continued for 6–12 months, and changes in cognitive function and mood, sleep and fatigue should be carefully monitored every 4–6 weeks during this time.

Clinical pearls

- Cognitive decline is a natural part of the ageing process and therefore needs to be managed, not cured.

- When diagnosing normal cognitive impairment it is important to rule out clinical depression.

- Medications have limited evidence, and lifestyle modification (physical and mental activity, social interaction and a wholefood healthy diet) is advised.

Expert | CONSULT

Clinical Comprehension Questions & Answers are hosted on
https://expertconsult.inkling.com/store/book/ sarris-clinical-naturopathy-case-files-1

BIBLIOGRAPHY

Essa MM, Vijayan RK, Castellano-Gonzalez G, et al. Neuroprotective effect of natural products against Alzheimer's disease. *Neurochem Res.* 2012;37(9):1829-1842.

Kure C. Ageing and cognition. In: Sarris J, Wardle J, eds. *Clinical Naturopathy: an Evidence-Based Guide to Practice*. 2nd ed. Australia: Churchill Livingstone; 2014.

Morley JE. Cognition and nutrition. *Curr Opin Clin Nutr Metab Care.* 2014;17(1):1-4.

Perry E, Howes MJR. Medicinal plants and dementia therapy: Herbal hopes for brain aging? *CNS Neurosci Ther.* 2011;17(6):683-698.

Varteresian T, Lavretsky H. Natural products and supplements for geriatric depression and cognitive disorders: an evaluation of the research. *Curr Psychiatry Rep.* 2014;16(8):1-9.

18 | Chronic fatigue syndrome

Stephanie Gadsden

PRESENTATION

A 25-year-old female presents with **ongoing chronic physical** and **mental fatigue** for the past 8 years. Previously a high achiever, she feels she **didn't completely recover from glandular fever** diagnosed at aged 16. She is unable to commit to full-time work or study, due to **recurring fatigue, low-grade inflammatory episodes**, a **sore throat, swollen lymph glands** and **headaches**. Twenty days in a month she is unable to get out of bed and **does not feel refreshed from sleep.** Short-term physical activity and mental exertion produces rebound fatigue. When fatigue is most severe (8/10), she complains of **aching legs, light headedness** and **dizziness**. Also diagnosed with **irritable bowel syndrome (IBS)** and multiple **food sensitivities and intolerances,** her diet is restricted and nutrient-poor. She feels increasingly **depressed** and overwhelmed with the limitations of her condition.

Diagnostic considerations

The pathophysiological abnormalities of chronic fatigue syndrome (CFS) suggest that CFS is a heterogeneous condition of complex and multifactorial aetiologies. Therefore treatment of the above case should involve an integrative approach acknowledging the mental, physical, environmental, emotional and spiritual elements of the condition.

As in this case, CFS can be associated with an infectious aetiology. Viral infections such as Epstein-Barr virus, human herpes virus 6 and enteroviruses are common precipitating factors. Other insults such as heavy metal exposure, mould and parasitic infection should be explored. It may be appropriate to recommend a home assessment to identify aggravating environmental factors.

Non-specific inflammatory episodes can be preceded by psychological stress. Infections are also a known initiator of CFS and, when involving the nervous system, contribute to depressive symptoms. A recommendation for this patient to engage in stress management in conjunction with immune support would be a crucial step in her rehabilitation.

It is important to differentiate CFS from clinical depression. Referral to a psychologist may be warranted for assessment and psychological support. As with this case, gut inflammation and IBS frequently parallels CFS. Gut health should be a primary focus of treatment, remembering that a well-functioning digestive system is integral to a healthy immune system. Her aching muscles could warrant investigations into fibromyalgia. Referral to manual therapies such as acupuncture and massage may be of benefit as well as supplementation with vitamin D.

Symptoms of light headiness and dizziness may indicate postural hypertension, which can be diagnosed with the tilt table test. Her restricted diet and poor nutrient intake may be contributing to CFS, involving deficiencies of nutrients such as zinc, coenzyme Q10 (co-Q10) and omega-3 polyunsaturated fatty acids.

COMMON MEDICAL CONDITIONS THAT MAY MIMIC OR OCCUR ALONGSIDE CHRONIC FATIGUE SYNDROME
- Clinical depression
- Fibromyalgia
- Adrenal disease
- Alcohol abuse
- Malignancy
- Sleep disorders
- Thyroid abnormalities
- Schizophrenia
- Anaemias

Treatment protocol

- Improve immune function and reduce inflammatory mediators by eliminating residual infections and inflammatory triggers. Herbs with antiviral, antimicrobial and anti-inflammatory properties include *Andrographis paniculata*, *Thymus vulgaris*, *Calendula officinalis*, *Curcuma longa* and *Echinacea purpurea*.

- Suggest psychological support with cognitive behaviour therapy (CBT) by referral to a psychologist or reputable online CBT course. Prescribe *Hypericum perforatum* for its combined hypothesised antiviral and antidepressant action.

- Assess for nutrient deficiencies and increased requirements to support mitochondrial function and combat oxidative stress by prescribing zinc, co-Q10, acetylcarnitine, oral D-ribose, magnesium and B vitamins. Injectable nutrients may be used if absorption is compromised. Implement a wholefood, balanced diet that is sufficient in protein, essential fatty acids, complex carbohydrates, fruits and vegetables.

- Restore the gastrointestinal tract with glutamine and probiotics (if necessary—and tailor to the patient's microbiota requirements). Digestive enzymes are effective in improving nutrient absorption and assimilation and to digest proteins contributing to a defective immune response. Assess for pathogenic overgrowth.

PRESCRIPTION
PHASE 1: ACUTE IMMUNE TREATMENT
Herbal formula (100 mL)

Andrographis paniculata 1:2	30 mL
Hypericum perforatum 1:2	30 mL
Echinacea root blend* 1:2	20 mL
Calendula officinalis 1:2	20 mL
Dose: 5 mL 3 × daily	

Herbal tablet

Curcuma longa: 2 g/day

PHASE 2: RESTORATIVE TREATMENT
Herbal formula (100 mL)

Eleutherococcus senticosus 1:2	30 mL
Rehmannia glutinosa 1:2	30 mL
Hypericum perforatum 1:2	25 mL
Glycyrrhiza glabra 1:1	15 mL
Dose: 5 mL 3 × daily	

Nutritional prescription

Zinc picolinate or citrate: 30 mg/day
Co-Q10: 150 mg/day
Magnesium citrate: 500 mg 3 × daily
Glutamine powder: 4.5 g 2 × daily

Lifestyle prescription

CBT and psychological support
Regular massage therapy
Graded exercise

E. purpurea 60%, *E. angustifolia* 40%

- Improve physical conditioning by incorporating graded exercise techniques co-supported with adaptogen herbs such as *Eleutherococcus senticosus*, *Panax ginseng*, *Withania somnifera* and *Rehmannia glutinosa*. Address postural hypertension by increasing fluids and sodium intake while supporting the adrenals and venous tone with herbs such as *Glycyrrhiza glabra* and *Aesculus hippocastanum*.

Expected outcomes and follow-up protocols

The patient should be made aware that CFS is a chronic condition that may take months to resolve. It is essential to engage a team of professionals to address all the needs of the patient—often simultaneously. Such team members include a psychologist, exercise physiologist, physiotherapist, nutritionist, massage therapist, acupuncturist and a physician.

It is important to initially restore immunological functioning. Management of external insults and by decreasing inflammation can help to improve recurrent lymphatic episodes alongside correcting gastrointestinal tract functioning. Practitioners can then aim to improve physical conditioning with nutrient therapy, adaptogenic herbs and graded exercise. It would be appropriate to recommend that she consult with an exercise physician to manage her activity levels.

Ongoing psychological support is essential, as is a recommendation for her to engage in stress management techniques and become aware of her limitations to prevent relapse. The patient should see a gradual improvement in fatigue and resolution of symptoms within 6–12 months; however, self-monitoring of triggers such as stress, toxicant exposure and food sensitivities is ongoing.

Clinical pearls

- Identify and manage key insults to the body from infection, environmental toxicants and psychological stress.

- When diagnosing CFS it is important to rule out other medical diagnoses such as iron deficiency or anaemia, thyroid abnormalities, sleep disorders, general fatigue and adrenal disease.

- If muscle and joint pain is present, this may warrant a diagnosis of fibromyalgia. Diagnostic criteria for fibromyalgia includes bilateral and multiple sites of trigger point pain, and must be differentiated from CFS.

Expert | CONSULT

Clinical Comprehension Questions & Answers are hosted on
https://expertconsult.inkling.com/store/book/
sarris-clinical-naturopathy-case-files-1

BIBLIOGRAPHY

Brown BI. Chronic fatigue syndrome: a personalized integrative medicine approach. *Altern Ther Health Med.* 2014;20(1):29-40.

Gadsden S, Deed G. *Chronic Fatigue Syndrome Clinical Naturopathy: An Evidence-Based Guide to Practice.* J. Sarris and J. Wardle. ed 2. Sydney: Elsevier; 2014.

Griffith JP, Zarrouf AA. Systemic review of chronic fatigue syndrome: don't assume it's depression. *Prim Care Companion J Clin Psychiatry.* 2008;10(2):120-128.

Lorusso L, Mikhaylova SV, Capelli E, et al. Immunological aspects of chronic fatigue syndrome. *Autoimmun Rev.* 2009;8(4):287-291.

Sarris J. *Depression. Clinical Naturopathy: An Evidence-Based Guide to Practice.* J. Sarris and J. Wardle. ed 2. Sydney: Elsevier; 2014:769-788.

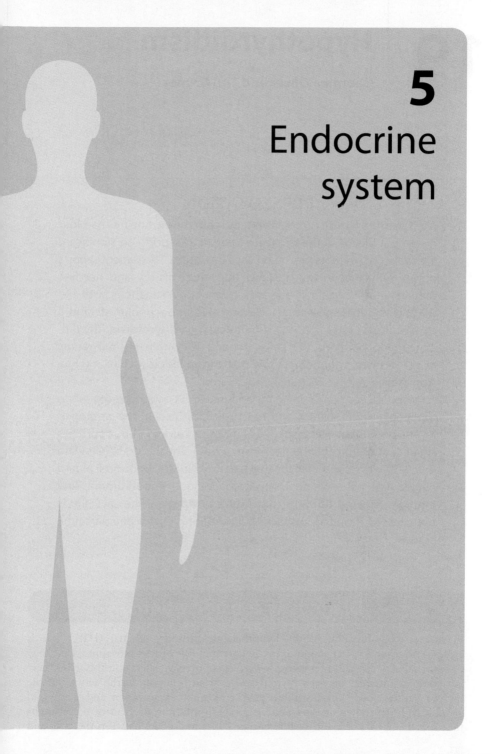

5
Endocrine system

19 | Hypothyroidism

Georgina Oliver and Tini Gruner

PRESENTATION

A 21-year-old female presents with **amenorrhoea**. She has had four menstrual bleeds in the last three years and reports no significant life events or stressors preceding their cessation. The patient reports no abnormalities in her previous menstrual history and her first menarche at 12 years of age was normal. Investigations with her GP and multiple specialists, including two endocrinologists and a gynaecologist, have revealed **subclinical hypothyroidism** (thyroid-stimulating hormone (TSH) 6.4, T4 and T3 within normal range, negative thyroid antibodies), **low oestrogen levels** (< 100) and **low iron stores** (ferritin 20, transferrin 36, iron 24, Hb 13.7).

Magnetic resonance imaging and pelvic ultrasound revealed no functional abnormalities and her prolactin, insulin and androgen levels are normal. Her body mass index is 22, and she reports no significant weight change since high school. She has been following a vegan, wholefood diet for the past 5 years for both ethical and health reasons. Additional symptoms include **hypersomnia**, **low energy**, **reduced libido**, **irritability** and **apathy**. She says she is not stressed, despite a busy schedule of full-time work and part-time study.

Diagnostic considerations

In this case, dysfunction of the hypothalamic–pituitary–adrenal (HPA) axis is evident. Additional investigations into the potential role of stress are appropriate (e.g. 24-hour salivary cortisol, rT3 levels), given its suppressive effects on this axis. There is a complex interplay between thyroid and ovarian function, as the activity of the thyroid gland is closely linked with the process of ovarian maturation, and the thyroid gland itself is dependent on direct and indirect stimuli from the ovaries to execute its function. It may be difficult to differentiate cause and effect between the two, and treatment should therefore be directed towards correcting hypothalamic–pituitary function.

Underlying medical conditions that may influence hypothalamic–pituitary or thyroid function directly—such as high cortisol levels, pituitary/thyroid tumours, hyperprolactinaemia and the use of certain medications such as lithium and interferon alpha—need to be investigated to exclude for secondary causes of hypothyroidism and amenorrhoea. Further, heavy metals such as mercury, lead and cadmium and environmental pollutants such as dioxins, furans and polychlorinated biphenyls have been found to disrupt endocrine function. The potential of these toxicities can be considered and detoxification strategies implemented as needed.

The World Health Organization suggests that iodine status is the most immediate measure of whether the thyroid gland has adequate iodine to function normally, therefore assessment of iodine levels through a urine sample may be valuable. Spot testing (random sample, not first-morning sample) may be more practical for patients to complete rather than 24-hour urine collection methods and appears adequate to detect iodine deficiency (so long as creatinine levels are also determined, which will account for the dilution of the random sample). However, in the absence of iodised salt and seaweed in a vegan diet, it is likely that an iodine deficiency would exist and supplementation will be necessary. Daily doses of iodine between 150 mcg and 300 mcg are suitable (doses greater than 500 mcg can inhibit thyroid function), and supplementation can be reduced to the recommended 150 mcg and adjusted for dietary intake once thyroid function is restored (evident through blood tests, ideally repeated every 3 months). Enquiry into any changes in the patient's weight is appropriate, given that amenorrhoea can occur as a result of low bodyweight and, conversely, hypothyroidism can reduce basal metabolic rate and lead to weight gain. If the patient is sexually active, appropriate contraception methods still need to be employed if pregnancy is undesired, and regular pregnancy tests should be conducted to exclude this as the cause of amenorrhoea.

Despite the many health benefits of a wholefood vegan diet, it can be at risk of various nutrient deficiencies, which may contribute to poor thyroid function and disturbances in the menstrual cycle—specifically, low vitamin D, iron, zinc, tyrosine and iodine. Low cholesterol levels may also be a concern given the low saturated fat and high fibre content of this diet. Nutrient absorption may be further compromised due to underlying malabsorption conditions such as coeliac disease or inflammatory bowel disease. Comprehensive questioning into digestive health and functioning of your patient will be required.

IMPORTANT DIAGNOSTIC/CLINICAL CONSIDERATIONS
- Hashimoto's thyroiditis
- Medications e.g. lithium, interferon alpha, antiarrhythmia medications
- Premature ovarian failure
- Nutrient deficiencies—particularly iodine, iron and/or vitamin D
- Heavy metal toxicities
- Environmental pollutants
- Hyperprolactinaemia
- Pituitary/thyroid tumour
- Pregnancy
- Coeliac disease
- Inflammatory bowel disease
- Polycystic ovary syndrome
- Low bodyweight
- Eating disorders
- Excessive exercise
- Low body mass index
- Depression
- Anxiety

Treatment protocol

- Ensure the diet contains nutrients required to facilitate healthy thyroid and ovarian function as well as supporting stress adaptation. Adequate dietary protein is required for sufficient tyrosine, and in vegan/vegetarian cases, varying protein sources across the day to provide complete proteins should be advised (legumes, whole grains, nuts and seeds).

- Goitrogenic foods (soy, brassicas, millet) should be cooked, and traditional sources of soy are preferred such as tempeh and miso paste. Iron-rich foods are essential given iron's role in ovulation and thyroid hormone production and to counteract the suppressive effects of low thyroid function on haematopoiesis. Seaweed is one of the best dietary sources of iodine, as well as iodised salt used in cooking. Kelp tablets may be appropriate if seaweed is not preferred.

- Ensure moderate amounts of saturated fats are included in the diet to provide dietary cholesterol, which may assist in hormone production and maintaining healthy menstrual cycles. Commend and encourage the patient to continue with her wholefood diet, as diets consisting predominantly of highly refined and processed foods may contribute to abnormal levels of inflammation and, therefore, disturb HPA activity and subsequently interfere with hormone production and function.

- *Vitex agnus-castus* can be used to assist in normalising pituitary function and is also beneficial for correcting luteal phase defects. In addition, a clinical study has highlighted its ability to increase progesterone and beta-oestradiol levels.

- *Withania somnifera* is a potential therapeutic option, given its ability to improve stress adaptation, lower cortisol and increase T3 and T4 levels. More recently, a case report within a randomised controlled trial involving people with bipolar disorder demonstrated normalising of TSH levels after 8 weeks of *Withania somnifera* supplementation.

- *Bacopa monnieri* increases T4 levels and possesses adaptogenic properties. Additional adaptogens and nervine tonics may be of benefit to relieve irritability, lower cortisol and improve energy. Consider *Lavandula angustifolia*, *Verbena officinalis*, *Scutellaria lateriflora*, *Rhodiola rosea*, *Panax ginseng* and/or *Eleutherococcus senticosus*.

- A vegan calcium supplement with cofactors required for bone health is warranted given oestrogen's role in bone mineral density and the low levels of oestrogen present in this case. Calcium may also assist in oocyte formation and the production of cervical mucus. Education regarding good sources of calcium in a vegan diet is also important. Consider a vegan vitamin D supplement for bone mineral density and hormone production if sun exposure to the skin is suspected to be inadequate.

- Exercise is key for improving stress adaptation and increasing the metabolic rate; however, caution needs to be taken to avoid excessive fat loss, which may further inhibit ovulation. Yoga is particularly beneficial for its cortisol-lowering effects. Certain poses are considered to be specific for improving hypothalamic function (e.g. shoulderstand and bow pose). Interval training is of benefit for improving the metabolic rate, energy levels and resilience to stress. Weight-bearing exercise is important to encourage bone mineral density.

- A mood and symptom diary may be helpful in determining menstrual cycle patterns such as breast tenderness, cycles of irritability/mood disturbances, food cravings, bloating and cervical mucus.

- Recording morning body temperature, taken with a thermometer at the same time before getting out of bed, can be utilised to monitor thyroid function and the occurrence of ovulation. This also reduces the reliance on frequent blood tests, which can become cumbersome and stressful in itself for the patient.

PRESCRIPTION

Herbal formula

Vitex agnus-castus (180 mg): 1 tablet (traditionally upon rising)

Nutritional prescription
Iron supplementation

Iron amino acid chelate/biglycinate (approx. 20 mg) with vitamin B6 and B12 and vitamin C cofactors required for RBC production and iron absorption: 1 tablet with breakfast

Vegetarian calcium supplement (powder) with cofactors (magnesium, phosphorus, boron, selenium, zinc, copper, sulphur, iodine): 1 tsp in water before the evening meal

Thyroid/adrenal complex

Tyrosine: 500 mg

Zinc citrate 12.5 equiv. zinc: 4 mg

Selenomethionine equiv. selenium: 50 mcg

Potassium iodide equiv. iodine: 100 mcg and equiv. potassium 30 mcg

Rehmannia glutinosa root ext. dry conc. equiv. rehmannia root dry: 400 mg

Withania somnifera root ext. dry conc. equiv. withania root dry: 300 mg

Thiamine hydrochloride: 10 mg

Riboflavin: 10 mg

Pyridoxine hydrochloride: 25 mg

equiv. pyridoxine: 20.5 mg

Nicotinic acid: 10 mg

Nicotinamide: 40 mg

Calcium pantothenate: 50 mg

equiv. pantothenic acid: 45.7 mg

Ascorbic acid: 100 mg

Chromium nicotinate: 143 mcg

equiv. chromium: 15 mcg

1 tablet 2 × daily 1 hour before meals

Lifestyle prescription

Exercise: yoga, weight training, interval training

Daily symptom and mood diary

Taking morning body temperature as much as possible for at least 3 months

Expected outcomes and follow-up protocols

Restoration of the hypothalamic–pituitary axis can take time, therefore encouragement to adhere to treatment is important in the absence of immediate symptom improvement. Monitor your patient for thyroid 'switching', as periods of hyperthyroidism can occur in patients with hypothyroidism, particularly in cases where thyroid antibodies are present. If so, treatment protocols will need to be adjusted accordingly, for example, reducing iodine levels and providing additional antioxidants to counteract heightened metabolism. However, management and support of stress is typically required in all abnormal thyroid cases.

If menstruation has not returned after 3 months of consistent *Vitex* supplementation, consider reassessing the patient's sex and thyroid hormone levels to gauge effects of treatment. Additional herbal medicines containing steroidal saponins such as *Asparagus racemosus* and/or *Tribulus terrestris* may be of benefit due to their effect on steroidogenesis. Endometrial tonics such as *Angelica sinensis* can be incorporated to assist in the proliferation of healthy endometrial tissue, which is delayed in hypo-oestrogenic states. Consider a referral to a psychologist or counsellor if psycho-emotional strain is evident and not responding adequately to naturopathic treatment.

Clinical pearls

- Be aware that thyroid conditions may oscillate between 'hyper' and 'hypo', particularly in cases where thyroid antibodies are present, therefore regular monitoring of TSH and T3/T4 levels is advised.

- 'Stress' may not always be described by the patient despite clear signs of stress affecting physiological functioning.

- Ensure all necessary medical investigations have been performed to exclude for underlying medical conditions contributing to presenting symptoms.

- Hypothyroidism does not always present with weight gain or other metabolic abnormalities such as disturbed glucose metabolism or high cholesterol.

Expert | CONSULT

Clinical Comprehension Questions & Answers are hosted on
**https://expertconsult.inkling.com/store/book/
sarris-clinical-naturopathy-case-files-1**

BIBLIOGRAPHY

Frodl T, O'Keane V. How does the brain deal with cumulative stress? A review with focus on developmental stress, HPA axis function and hippocampal structure in humans. *Neurobiol Dis*. 2013;52:24-37.

Gruner T. Thyroid abnormalities. In: Sarris J, Wardle J, eds. *Clinical Naturopathy: An Evidence-Based Guide to Practice*. Sydney: Churchill Livingstone; 2014.

Ravanbod M, Asadipooya K, Kalantarhormozi M, et al. Treatment of iron-deficiency anemia in patients with subclinical hypothyroidism. *Am J Med*. 2013;126(5):420-424.

Van Die MD, Burger HG, Teede HJ, et al. *Vitex agnus-castus* extracts for female reproductive disorders: a systematic review of clinical trials. *Planta Med*. 2013;79(7):562-575.

Walter KN, Corwin EJ, Ulbrecht J, et al. Elevated thyroid-stimulating hormone is associated with elevated cortisol in healthy young men and women. *Thyroid Res*. 2012;5(1):1-6.

20 | Generalised stress and fatigue

Jerome Sarris and Tini Gruner

PRESENTATION

A 45-year-old female presents with **gradual onset of pronounced tiredness** over the past year. She had been working very long hours for several years in a corporate enterprise while also raising two children. She quit her job due to debilitating fatigue, but weeks later her energy levels are still very low. The patient **sleeps from 8 pm and wakes at 6.30 am unrefreshed**. She feels there is **less enjoyment in her life** and says **she can't concentrate** (tends to forget even routine activities). She **craves sweet and starchy foods** (eats a low-protein diet) and **drinks 4–6 cups of coffee a day** with minimal benefit. A psychiatric assessment has ruled out major depressive disorder, and medical tests have not revealed any major pathology. Her specialist does not believe she has chronic fatigue syndrome.

Diagnostic considerations

This patient has been exposed to a number of stressors over a long time including a demanding job and raising children. She has used stimulants, such as coffee, and carbohydrate-rich foods in order to increase adrenal output and maintain energy levels. While this approach did assist her initially, it has lost effect over time. Presentations such as these often point towards the potential for an endocrine disorder; however, sometimes no frank pathology exists, and the experience of 'chronic generalised fatigue' may be due to general neuroendocrine dysfunction from an excessive allostatic load. This has been previously coined in naturopathy as 'adrenal exhaustion', which while not being a medical diagnosis as such, reflects the exhaustion phase of the generalised adaptation syndrome (GAS) scale. The diagnosis of being in the exhaustion phase of the GAS scale may be confirmed via salivary tests revealing low cortisol in both the morning (where it has meant to have peaked) persisting into the afternoon and evening. Blood tests may also reveal low levels of one-carbon cycle factors that assist in the methylation process (e.g. folate, B12, SAMe). While theoretically it is possible to test for urinary metabolites of neurotransmitters involved with energy production and mood, there is currently no evidence validating such techniques or their direct relation to medical disorders. A blood test may also be considered to test the status of other nutrient deficiencies that may be affecting her energy levels.

Other traditional diagnostic techniques such as pulse and tongue assessment (while not medically validated) may assist in establishing she is in the exhaustion phase. A pulse that is weak or slow and a tongue that is pale and flabby may indicate this, as opposed to the presentation of a rapid strong pulse and red tongue. In such cases the person may present with fatigue; however, it may be due to a latent postviral infection or increased cortisol levels (which may present as fatigue with an overlay of perceived stress and a sense of being hyped yet fatigued and 'running on empty'). Medical tests are critical to rule out any pathological causation (e.g. cancer, thyroid dysfunction, Addison's disease) in addition to psychological assessment for major depressive disorder (or bipolar disorder).

IMPORTANT DIAGNOSTIC/CLINICAL CONSIDERATIONS

- Chart a history of energy and stress levels, allostatic load factors and key stressors
- Screen for mood or anxiety disorders
- Consider thyroid dysfunction or any underlying endocrine pathology
- Rule out any pathogenic influences, chronic fatigue syndrome or fibromyalgia
- Screen/refer for cognitive decline/early dementia
- Monitor stimulant and alcohol misuse

Treatment protocol

- The herbal prescription is designed primarily to enhance her energy via the use of adaptogens and stimulating traditional 'tonics'. *Rhodiola rosea* and *Panax ginseng* will provide this, in addition to the formula being augmented by *Glycyrrhiza glabra* to increase cortisol levels.

- Because she complains of feeling cold and having poor circulation, *Zingiber officinale* may be beneficial as a warming circulatory stimulant. *Bacopa monnieri* is prescribed to assist with improving the 'memory' cognitive domain.

- Coenzyme Q10 (co-Q10) is prescribed for assistance with energy production in the electron transport chain. A multivitamin may address any underlying nutrient deficiencies, while the B vitamins are beneficial to assist in energy production and allay fatigue, being critical in the proper function of the energy cycle. Zinc and magnesium are key minerals required in many enzymatic processes critical for proper neuroendocrine function.

- In respect of addressing her lifestyle, she is advised to eat more protein, as this is critical for the production of key enzymes and neurotransmitters.

Other lifestyle advice involves recommending graduated exercise to build her stamina and improve her energy levels. Teaching breathing techniques may also provide relaxation as well as improving general vigour. Removing or reducing caffeine is a vital component to provide less stimulation of adrenergic activity while she is in convalescence.

PRESCRIPTION
Herbal formula (100 mL)

Rhodiola rosea 1:2	45 mL
Panax ginseng 1:2	30 mL
Glycyrrhiza glabra 1.2	20 mL
Zingiber officinale 1:2	5 mL

Dose: 5 mL in the morning and 5 mL after lunch

Bacopa monnieri: 1 tablet 2 × daily

Nutritional prescription

Co-Q10: 100 mg/day

Multivitamin high in B vitamins, zinc and magnesium: 1 tablet 2 × daily

Lifestyle prescription

Graduated exercise

Breathing techniques

Reduced caffeine

Increased protein in the diet

Expected outcomes and follow-up protocols

With such a 'tonifying' prescription, an increase in energy is expected within a couple of weeks. Depending on the level of exhaustion (i.e. depending on the duration and intensity of the allostatic load), it may take longer to build vitality. Regardless, there is still scope for changing the treatment should the current prescription fail to produce the desired results (e.g. improved mood, energy and coping ability). If no effect is seen within 1 month, then further referral may be needed, and/or the potential to increase the co-Q10 dosage, or modification of the prescription with thymoleptics such as S-adenosylmethionine or *Hypericum perforatum* (if mood issues are considered to be a crucial factor). Another consideration is referral for a glucose tolerance test to see whether there are any glucose or insulin function abnormalities.

In the current case, as both physical and mental/emotional symptoms are present, this needs to be taken into consideration in the design of a treatment plan. The connection between psychological, neurological and endocrine symptoms is now well established in disciplines such as psychoneuroendocrinology. In longer standing problems (as is the case in chronic fatigue), cellular metabolism is often further compromised, with potential oxidative damage to the neurological system potentially leading to the development of a range of chronic diseases. Treatment in that case would be advised to be more comprehensive and extended over a longer time span. Allostatic load can be modified and reduced, and a positive mental attitude, a purpose in life and a pursuit of personal growth may be of assistance. Achieving a good nutritional status and a balanced lifestyle is important and needs to be the core of addressing patients with chronic stress and fatigue.

Clinical pearls

- Stress activates the hypothalamus–pituitary–adrenal axis and triggers the release of a cascade of hormones and neurotransmitters, notably adrenalin and cortisol.

- With prolonged stress this may lead to a gradual decline of adrenal function and neurotransmitters, and finally to a state of psychophysiological exhaustion.

- Practitioners need to discern between the alarm, adaptation and exhaustion phases and test for the presence of either high or low cortisol levels.

- Treatment needs to focus on both the physical and the mental/emotional aspects of stress.

Expert | CONSULT

Clinical Comprehension Questions & Answers are hosted on **https://expertconsult.inkling.com/store/book/ sarris-clinical-naturopathy-case-files-1**

BIBLIOGRAPHY

Eidelman D. Fatigue: towards an analysis and a unified definition. *Med Hypotheses.* 1980;6(5):517-526.

Gruner T, Sarris J. Stress and fatigue. In: Sarris J, Wardle J, eds. *Clinical Naturopathy: An Evidence-Based Guide to Practice.* 2nd ed. Australia: Churchill Livingstone; 2014.

Panossian A, Wikman G. Evidence-based efficacy of adaptogens in fatigue, and molecular mechanisms related to their stress-protective activity. *Curr Clin Pharmacol.* 2009;4(3):198-219.

Panossian A, Wikman G, Sarris J. Rosenroot (*Rhodiola rosea*): traditional use, chemical composition, pharmacology and clinical efficacy. *Phytomedicine.* 2010;17(7):481-493.

21 Metabolic syndrome

Georgina Oliver and Tini Gruner

PRESENTATION

A 58-year-old male presents with **poor sleep, low energy, shortness of breath** and **headaches**. With further questioning, he reports **high levels of stress** from his work environment, which is predominantly sedentary in nature, as well as ongoing conflict within his family. His **diet is high in processed 'convenience' foods**, particularly fried foods, and he reports not enjoying cooking because he lives on his own. Despite being fit in his early adulthood, he reports he is now 'too busy to exercise'. He carries **excess abdominal weight** (waist circumference 125 cm) and has thin arms and legs. Recent investigations with his GP revealed **high blood glucose** (7.5 nmol/L), **high blood pressure** (150/110) and **elevated triglycerides** (2.5 nmol/L), and therefore he has been diagnosed with **metabolic syndrome**.

Diagnostic considerations

Metabolic syndrome is a major risk factor for developing diabetes, cardiovascular disease and chronic kidney disease. Therefore preventing the progression of metabolic syndrome is key in this case.

The diagnosis of metabolic syndrome may account for the majority of the patient's presenting symptoms and guides an immediate treatment protocol. However, consideration of other medical conditions is important. The possibility of sleep apnoea needs to be excluded, given the main presenting complaints of poor sleep, low energy and headaches. Thyroid function, vitamin D levels, cortisol and homocysteine investigations may also highlight contributing factors and provide additional treatment guidelines.

Further questioning into stress, mood and anxiety is necessary to ascertain underlying mental health conditions that commonly present with metabolic syndrome. Further medical tests may be required to rule out any cardiovascular conditions and to monitor the metabolic syndrome.

IMPORTANT DIAGNOSTIC/CLINICAL CONSIDERATIONS
- Sleep apnoea
- Generalised anxiety disorder
- Hypothyroidism
- Angina
- Major depressive disorder
- Cushing's syndrome
- Asthma
- Pneumonia
- Anaemia

Treatment protocol

- Patient education regarding the effects and consequences of metabolic syndrome is essential for the patient to identify the underlying causes of his presenting symptoms and encourage motivation for necessary changes in his diet and lifestyle. As lifestyle factors, rather than medication, are considered first-line treatments for metabolic syndrome, this too should be emphasised to the patient to encourage adherence to your treatment protocol.

- Metabolic syndrome often resides with substantial inflammation and oxidative stress, which is believed to exacerbate and sustain the condition. This can often be the effects of chronic, elevated cortisol levels due to poorly resolved psychological or physical stressors. Treatment to both indirectly (fat loss, blood glucose regulation) and directly (anti-inflammatory and antioxidant herbs, nutrients, dietary components and exercise strategies) reduce these events is imperative.

- Exercise is paramount in the treatment and management of metabolic syndrome, as well as improving resilience to stress, energy and sleep. Time constraints are considered one of the largest reasons why adults do not achieve the recommended exercise targets for optimal health, therefore identifying strategies for patient adherence to exercise is vital. High-intensity interval training (HIIT) can be of particular benefit in those with metabolic syndrome due to its positive effects on increasing physical fitness (maximal oxygen uptake), improving insulin sensitivity, increasing visceral fat loss and its anti-inflammatory effects. HIIT is of particular benefit given the short time it takes to complete and achieve these outcomes. Group fitness classes, exercising with a friend or personal training sessions are some of the best ways to encourage patient compliance when recommencing exercise.

- Modifications to diet and eating habits are paramount; however, they are often the hardest for patients to implement and maintain. Again, the importance of these dietary changes and their positive benefits for alleviating the presenting complaints need to be emphasised. Several studies highlight the benefits of following a Mediterranean dietary pattern for metabolic syndrome as well as reducing the risk of subsequent diabetes and cardiovascular disease. Further, the higher the adherence to this style of diet, the greater the health outcomes. The Mediterranean diet is particularly abundant in vegetables, fruits, legumes and whole grains and advocates regular consumption of fish, cultured dairy products and less meat. Together, this plant-based diet possesses a low glycaemic load, a feature that has also been found particularly beneficial for metabolic syndrome, diabetes and cardiovascular disease.

- Ensuring adequate protein and fibre is included at each meal will also assist in insulin sensitivity, appetite regulation and gut microbiota health, the latter largely responsible for modulating the inflammatory response. Limiting fried, processed and packaged foods is required to improve blood pressure (primarily through a reduction of sodium intake) and blood glucose levels. Increasing the content, and consuming a variety, of vegetables will provide the fibre and phytochemicals necessary for reducing triglyceride levels, improve blood glucose regulation and reduce oxidative stress and inflammation. Education regarding healthy eating-out options and exploring strategies of how more cooking can be done at home will also be important for long-term compliance. These dietary modifications may be gradual, therefore set small targets for the patient to implement to avoid them feeling overwhelmed.

- Poor sleep is considered a risk factor for weight gain and the development of metabolic syndrome. Ensuring good-quality sleep is necessary for improving energy, stress management, blood glucose regulation, lowering blood pressure and encouraging weight loss. Identifying a sleep hygiene routine for the patient and/or using a sleep/meditation app before bed may be useful.

- Levels of coenzyme Q10 (co-Q10) decline with age, and its cardioprotective activity will be of particular benefit in treating metabolic syndrome. Co-Q10 has been found to reduce blood glucose levels, blood pressure and triglyceride levels. In addition, its antioxidant activity protects against lipid peroxidation and therefore reduces cardiovascular complications such as atherosclerosis.

- Adaptogens can be used to improve carbohydrate metabolism, modulate cortisol level, improve stress resilience and alleviate anxiety. *Eleutherococcus senticosus* provides additional potential benefits for reducing blood pressure and triglyceride levels and improving glucose metabolism.

- Nutrients and herbal medicines to support glucose metabolism and provide additional antioxidant and anti-inflammatory activity such as zinc, chromium, lipoic acid, B vitamins, *Galega officinalis*, *Momordica charantia*, *Trigonella foenum-graecum* and *Gymnema sylvestre* are beneficial. Many tablet-based formulations for balancing blood glucose levels are available in varying combinations of the above list.

PRESCRIPTION

Herbal formula

Eleutherococcus senticosus (1:2)
Dose: 5 mL upon rising

Nutrient/herbal formula

Co-Q10 150 mg: 1 capsule in the morning with food
Zinc amino acid chelate 30 mg: 1 tablet with the evening meal

Herbal/nutrient formulation

Momordica charantia (equiv. 3 g fresh herb)
Galega officinalis (equiv. 2 g fresh herb)
Gymnema sylvestre leaf (equiv. 2 g dried herb)
Trigonella foenum-graecum (equiv. 400 mg dried herb)
R-, S-alpha-lipoic acid: 200 mg
Biotin: 1 mg
Chromium (as chloride): 250 mcg
Chromium (as picolinate): 50 mcg
Dose: 1 tablet 2 × daily with food

Lifestyle prescription

Exercise: High-intensity interval training/group fitness classes
Diet: Progressively implementing a Mediterranean dietary pattern; increasing vegetable intake, reducing processed and packaged foods; encouraging the patient to cook, as well as exploring healthy eating-out options
Sleep hygiene routine and/or meditation app

Expected outcomes and follow-up protocols

Core management of metabolic syndrome is implementing and adhering to healthy diet and lifestyle behaviours; however, these changes can often be the hardest for patients to implement and maintain. It is common to find that patients are unable to adopt the therapeutic strategies initially outlined. If so, find out what is practical and manageable for the patient, and ensure changes are made gradually for long-term sustainability. If diet and exercise recommendations are employed, improvement in energy and sleep can be reported in as little as 1 week. However, consistency is vital for long-term benefits and desirable changes in blood tests. Relapses are to be expected. Advising patients of this before they occur will mitigate their often perceived sense of failure and instead encourage the patient to learn from setbacks and continue with the outlined healthy behaviours.

It is important to review the blood tests used to assess the status of metabolic syndrome (triglycerides, cholesterol, fasting blood glucose) to ensure your treatment protocols are improving the condition. HbA_{1C} (glycated haemoglobin) can be used to provide a more sensitive measure of blood glucose status, as this gives an average of the amount of glucose in the bloodstream for the past 8–12 weeks rather than an acute morning reading determined by fasting glucose tests. Regular monitoring of weight and abdominal measurements are also advised; however, this needs to be handled delicately.

If headaches and shortness of breath do not alleviate with improvements in stress, sleep, fitness, blood glucose control and/or blood pressure readings, additional investigations will need to be conducted with a GP. Always check in with patients regarding their stress levels. As modulation of cortisol is essential for treating and managing metabolic syndrome, additional strategies may be required to improve stress management and sleep quality. Referral to a psychologist or a regular meditation-based practice may also be useful.

Clinical pearls

- Although nutritional supplements provide an important role in treating metabolic syndrome, the importance of dietary and lIfestyle factors should not be overlooked. These are the best long-term therapeutic agents and the most empowering tools for the patient.

- Patients can be motivated to implement treatment strategies once a 'formal' diagnosis has been made and awareness of its complications understood. Education as to how the condition can be treated and managed with diet, lifestyle, nutrients and/or herbal medicine can also be highly motivating for the patient.

- Anthropometrics are important for monitoring your patient's condition, rather than solely relying on their GP for blood tests. Recording regular waist circumference measurements is an easy and highly valuable monitor of metabolic syndrome status.

- Tailor diet and exercise recommendations to each patient, encouraging them to implement change but always working within their capabilities.

Expert | CONSULT

Clinical Comprehension Questions & Answers are hosted on https://expertconsult.inkling.com/store/book/ sarris-clinical-naturopathy-case-files-1

BIBLIOGRAPHY

Esser N, Legrand-Poels S, Piette J, et al. Inflammation as a link between obesity, metabolic syndrome and type 2 diabetes. *Diabetes Res Clin Pract.* 2014;105(2):141-150.

Gruner T. Type 2 diabetes and insulin resistance. In: Sarris J, Wardle J, eds. *Clinical Naturopathy: An Evidence-Based Guide to Practice.* 2nd ed. Australia: Churchill Livingstone; 2014.

Kastorini CM, Milionis HJ, Esposito K, et al. The effect of Mediterranean diet on metabolic syndrome and its components: a meta-analysis of 50 studies and 534,906 individuals. *J Am Coll Cardiol.* 2011;57(11):1299-1313.

Little JP, Gillen JB, Percival M, et al. Low-volume high-intensity interval training reduces hyperglycemia and increases muscle mitochondrial capacity in patients with type 2 diabetes. *J Appl Physiol.* 2011;111(6):1554-1560.

Royal Australian College of General Practice, Growing epidemics: the metabolic syndrome, http://www.racgp.org.au/afp/2013/august/the-metabolic-syndrome/#3.

Welty FK, Alfaddagh A, Elajami TK. Targeting inflammation in metabolic syndrome. *Transl Res.* 2015;167(1):257-280.

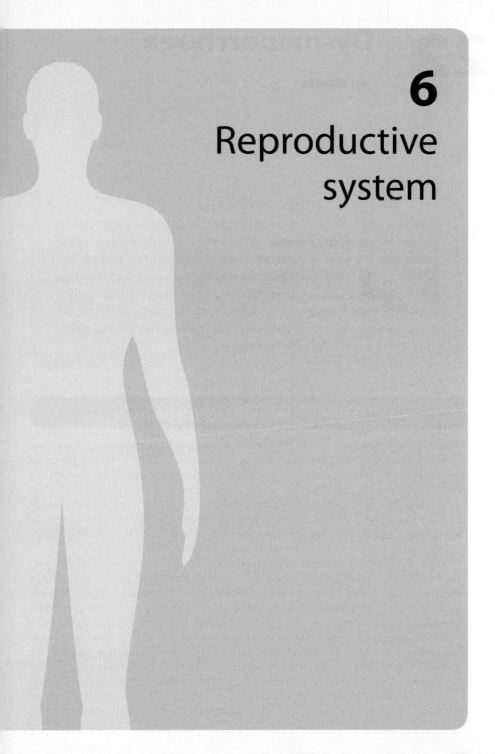

6
Reproductive system

22 Dysmenorrhoea

Jon Wardle

PRESENTATION

A 24-year-old female presents to the clinic complaining of intensely (spasmodic) **painful periods**, which she has experienced since menarche. The **pain is more noticeable towards the end of the period**. She says **she has tried everything, including naturopathy** and nothing has ever made a difference. She says she has 'regular bowel motions', which upon questioning are discovered to be approximately one every five days. The patient has an otherwise 'healthy' diet and exercises regularly.

Diagnostic considerations

Symptoms can often be entirely removed from the patient's presenting complaint. The main aim of naturopathic medicine is specifically to restore natural processes and, in doing so, the patient's health. When the patient is obviously aberrant (as bowel function is in this case), restoring normal functionality should be a major goal of naturopathic treatment. This case also highlights that even simple changes can elicit pronounced clinical results. It is always imperative that practitioners avoid 'over-treating' as much as they don't 'under-treat'. However, as this case highlights, it is important to address immediate concerns as well.

While naturopathic treatment does (and should) focus on uncovering the 'root cause' of symptoms, this is not often the driver of the initial patient visit. Initial treatment needs to focus on the patient's presenting concerns and adequately educate the patient as to the importance of the root cause in treatment of their condition, otherwise the patient may not comply with broader treatment goals. This case also helps to highlight the problematic element of language in the case-taking process. Patient and practitioner perceptions of 'regular' or 'normal' can differ. Specifics are required to adequately inform clinical practice. This patient highlighted a raft of therapies that had been ineffective, including most of the naturopathic armamentarium. It is unlikely that something that was previously ineffective will be effective without significant change in the patient, so eliminating previously ineffective treatments is vital to building an effective treatment. Asking about previous therapies can also help to uncover patterns; in this case it became apparent that previous practitioner focus on hormones and reproductive therapies was not working, and that the problem may lie elsewhere.

CONDITIONS THAT MAY MIMIC DYSMENORRHOEA SYMPTOMS

- Endometriosis
- Ovarian cysts
- Irritable bowel syndrome
- Inflammatory bowel disease
- Urinary tract infection
- Pelvic inflammatory disease

Treatment protocol

- Given the preponderance of previous failed treatments, immediate therapy is symptomatic, while underlying issues affecting the pain are explored. Consistent failure of previous treatments should serve as a red flag that similar approaches will not be successful.

- Symptomatic herbs include *Viburnum opulus* and *Corydalis ambigua*, which have strong traditional use as uterine relaxants via their spasmolytic action. This spasmolytic activity can be complemented with the analgesic activity of *Corydalis ambigua* and the anti-inflammatory activity of *Zingiber officinale*. It should be noted that this combination is effectively aimed at treating the symptoms of dysmenorrhoea and do not address its underlying cause. For this reason, they are only prescribed in the lead-up to, and the duration of, menses.

- The primary treatment rationale for herbal medicine treatment in this case is purely symptomatic—antispasmodic and anti-inflammatory to relieve menstrual cramping. This is done only to ensure patient compliance in treating the root cause of her symptoms, which can take some time.

- After the consultation process it became apparent that the patient had emotional issues attached to defecation. This was uncovered in her reaction to discussing the issue but confirmed upon further questioning. At this point the patient should be reassured that a symptomatic, but temporary, treatment for her immediate symptom is available (as prescribed). However, the patient also needs to be extensively counselled on the importance of bowel functions to normal body processes, as well as the 'normal' and cleansing aspects of it. This is an exhaustive and educative component of treatment, focusing not only on the condition but also on anatomical and physiological concepts more broadly, and highlights the importance of education as a part of a naturopathic therapist's approach.

PRESCRIPTION
Herbal formula

Tablet containing:

Viburnum opulus: 800 mg dry root

Corydalis ambigua: 1200 mg dry root

Zingiber officinale: 800 mg dry root

Taken only in the lead-up to and during menses: 1 tablet 3 × daily 3 days prior to the period and then 2 tablets 3–4 × daily for 3 days until menses ceases

Lifestyle prescription

Counselling and education on the natural role of defecation in maintaining health

Expected outcomes and follow-up protocols

Pain reduction is often the most commonly sought treatment in many reproductive disorders and is ordinarily one in which improvement will be seen rather quickly, if treatment is effective. Similarly, resolving underlying issues affecting pain can also occur quite quickly. However, what can take longer is getting patients to accept links between different body systems. In this case the patient was largely sceptical of any role that increasing defecation could have on reducing period pain. Prescribing a symptomatic formula was therefore done as much to elicit a short-term improvement in results and therefore positive patient attitude towards other aspects discussed in treatment as it was to address the patient's presenting complaint. This may prove to be important, especially if during a return visit the patient recounts how they doubted the advice given during the consultation, and only when the product provided relief did they have confidence in other advice given during the consult.

It is also important to realise that, in any counselling environment, challenging a patient's longstanding beliefs may make them uncomfortable. It is not a therapy that can be rushed or done in an environment that is not conducive to doing so. The patient had viewed defecation as a 'disgusting' act that needed to be performed as sparingly as possible for two decades, and this cannot be resolved in the last 10 minutes of a session. Such approaches need to be individualised, as people will respond differently. At all times, though, it requires a foundation of trust. Although it can be tempting to focus on educating the patient about how they should get better, if the patient is not being listened to in other areas (for example, symptomatic therapy), they are usually unable to continue receiving counselling or education.

Clinical pearls

- Menstrual problems are not associated with simple hormone excess or deficiency but rather a complex interconnection of factors that interfere with the HPO axis.

- Dysmenorrhoea can be a symptom of other underlying conditions, not just a condition in and of itself.

- Premenstrual syndrome symptoms are often treated successfully by ameliorating underlying causes with dietary and lifestyle modification— women were not designed to 'malfunction' once a month.

- Symptomatic treatment is very important. However, smooth muscle relaxants or analgesics should be considered only a temporary solution and treating the underlying factors should be prioritised.

- Treating primary dysmenorrhoea should see positive results within the first one or two cycles.

- Secondary dysmenorrhoea requires treatment of its causative aetiology and is often more complex.

- If treatments haven't worked previously, they are unlikely to work again.

- It is unlikely the patient would have taken the counselling on board if their presenting problem had not shown improvement. Do not focus on the underlying cause so much that you ignore addressing the patient's priority symptoms.

Expert | CONSULT

Clinical Comprehension Questions & Answers are hosted on
https://expertconsult.inkling.com/store/book/ sarris-clinical-naturopathy-case-files-1

BIBLIOGRAPHY

Altman G, Jarrett MF, Burr RL, et al. Increased symptoms in female IBS patients with dysmenorrhea and PMS. *Gastroenterol Nurs.* 2006;29(1):4-11.

de Vrese M. Health benefits of probiotics and prebiotics in women. *Menopause Int.* 2009;15(1):35-40.

Girman A, Lee R, Kligler B. An integrative medicine approach to premenstrual syndrome. *Am J Obstet Gynecol.* 2003;188(5 suppl):S56-S65.

Hudson T. *Women's Encyclopedia of Natural Medicine.* New York: McGraw-Hill; 2008.

Trickey R. *Women, Hormones and the Menstrual Cycle: Herbal and Medical Solutions From Adolescence to Menopause.* Melbourne: MHHG; 2012.

Wardle J. Dysmenorrhoea. In: Sarris J, Wardle J, eds. *Clinical Naturopathy: An Evidence-Based Guide to Practice.* Sydney: Churchill Livingstone; 2014.

23 Endometriosis and menorrhagia

Jon Wardle

PRESENTATION

A 24-year-old female presents to the clinic complaining of intensely **painful periods**, which she has experienced since menarche. The **pain is more noticeable towards the end of the period** and she also experiences pain in the middle of the cycle, albeit in differing areas (she points to upper and lower abdominal areas). **Her bleeding is heavy**, and she is often required to take an 'emergency bag' of sanitary products whenever she leaves her house during her period. She experiences daily **nausea, indigestion** and **flatulence**. She and her partner have been **trying unsuccessfully to fall pregnant** for the past 9 months and she has laparoscopically-confirmed endometriosis.

Diagnostic considerations

In naturopathic treatment, endometriosis is most often considered a disorder of hormonal imbalance (usually related to oestrogen) or inflammation and may have a number of underlying factors. The diagnostic process should aim to uncover which of these major factors may be most influential in the presentation. Oestrogen modulation is often a focus of naturopathic treatment and can be elicited via: treatments that work on the hypothalamic–pituitary–ovarian (HPO) axis; compounds (phyto-oestrogens) that mimic endogenous sex hormones; encouraging oestrogen excretion (mainly via the liver) and other detoxification pathways. Exploring the function of each of these areas can highlight if any of these should be prioritised in treatment.

Inflammation is also highly indicated in endometriosis, with some strong aetiological links between endometriosis and autoimmunity. Reducing inflammation can reduce adhesions and improve symptoms so should also form a focus of treatment. Dietary and lifestyle risk factors are present in endometriosis and attention should be drawn to these during treatment—they include lack of exercise (though strenuous exercise during menses can increase risk), increased carbohydrate consumption, stress, low body mass index, alcohol, tobacco and coffee. When treating patients for female reproductive disorders it is always important to ascertain whether they are currently trying to get pregnant. Some treatments may have adverse events for fertility, but even when they don't, they can be pharmacologically active enough to warrant caution. A healthy body is usually a fertile body, and resolving underlying reproductive health issues will ultimately assist the patient's goal of a healthy pregnancy better than acute treatment. It is important to also observe non-reproductive symptoms, particularly those with a high incidence in reproductive disorders (such as irritable bowel syndrome-type symptoms).

MEDICAL CONDITIONS THAT MAY MIMIC OR AGGRAVATE ENDOMETRIOSIS SYMPTOMS

- Primary or secondary dysmenorrhoea
- Benign or malignant neoplasms (both gynaecological and non-gynaecological)
- Pelvic inflammatory disease
- Appendicitis
- Urinary tract infections
- Venereal diseases

Treatment protocol

- The primary rationale for herbal medicine treatment is regulating hormone feedback and production mechanisms via *Vitex agnus-castus* and *Actaea/Cimicifuga racemosa* to modulate hormone levels through their various mechanisms, as they may help restore proper functioning of the HPO axis through direct and indirect means.

- A traditionally focused reproductive-specific treatment approach is employed for symptomatic relief. The treatment rationale is antispasmodic (*Achillea millefolium* and *Viburnum opulus*), antihaemorrhagic (*Achillea millefolium*) and anti-inflammatory (*Glycyrrhiza glabra*). This is used to complement therapies with a more established evidence base.

- A 'maintenance' herbal formula is prescribed and should be taken throughout the month for hormone modulation. Changes may be appropriate during menses if the treatment does not take effect.

- Her dietary recommendations also focus on modulating hormones (namely oestrogen), both through increasing excretion through specific liver pathways and by using selective oestrogen receptor-modulating foods.

- With the autoimmune-like parameters observed in endometriosis, anti-inflammatory therapy is a primary consideration. Vitamin D and vitamin A are in part prescribed to address this. Developing a beneficial environment for appropriate intestinal microbial populations should be encouraged with fermented foods and the prebiotic soluble fibre *Ulmus rubra*.

- Lifestyle changes that discourage inflammation-mediating hormonal factors are advised including therapies that increase fitness, improve sleep and reduce stress. Foods that are known to aggravate the condition are recommended to be removed.

PRESCRIPTION
Herbal formula (100 mL)

Viburnum opulus 1:2	30 mL
Achillea millefolium 1:2	20 mL
Glycyrrhiza glabra 1:2	20 mL
Actaea/Cimicifuga racemosa 1:2	20 mL
Vitex agnus-castus 1:2	10 mL

Dose: 5 mL 3 × daily

Ulmus rubra bark powder: 10 g at night

Nutritional prescription

Vitamin D: 1300 IU/day (via cod liver oil—1 tbsp, which also contains 13,000 IU vitamin A)

Lifestyle prescription

Moderate balanced exercise: qi gong

Good sleep hygiene and mindfulness meditation

Dietary improvement including specific increases of cruciferous foods, phyto-oestrogen-rich foods and fermented foods

Iron levels are monitored and the patient advised to eat iron-rich foods, with supplementation if iron levels become depleted through heavy menstrual flow

Expected outcomes and follow-up protocols

Pain reduction is often the most commonly sought treatment in many reproductive disorders. Although resolving underlying health issues is clearly important, patients will be less compliant if no progress is made in these acute symptoms. With acute naturopathic treatment, initial signs of improvement should be noticed within the first or second menses if it is likely to be effective. Persisting with a therapy that adequately resolves underlying issues but doesn't effectively address immediate symptoms will neither meet the patient's needs nor encourage them to continue with treatment. In endometriosis, although infertility is a common side effect, pregnancy itself can be more effective in reducing growths than conventional or naturopathic treatment. If the patient is attempting to get pregnant, the focus should be on moving away from contraindicated therapies, even if these are required in the initial stages for symptomatic relief.

Dietary and lifestyle factors cannot only effectively manage many symptoms but also improve the effectiveness of other treatments. Noticeable improvement should occur by the second cycle, providing dietary and lifestyle changes are also addressed. This should be especially noticeable in terms of abdominal pain, bloating and concomitant gastrointestinal symptoms. Women with larger or more ingrained endometrial growths will require oestrogen-modulating and anti-inflammatory treatment for some months to reduce and remove well-established endometrial growths, particularly those in 'enclosed' or 'removed' areas—such as those in areas not commonly associated with menstrual flow (for example, the intestines and kidneys). Patients should be notified that this could take up to 12 months or more in difficult cases, and that results are extremely variable between patients.

Clinical pearls

- Endometriosis shares many properties with autoimmune conditions. Examine the inflammatory status of the patient, and do not rely on hormonal modulation alone.

- Endometriosis is an oestrogen-dependent condition. Look at the factors that may influence this, including liver function, HPO function and nervous system function.

- Endometriosis is a complex condition with many interconnecting systems. It is likely that the condition is multifactorial and a number of treatment approaches are required. Do not fall into the temptation of over-focusing on one factor (such as hormones).

- Many of these factors have underlying nutritional or lifestyle aetiologies. Do not overcomplicate things. Studies suggest that sometimes simple dietary modifications may be enough to significantly improve outcomes.

Expert | CONSULT

Clinical Comprehension Questions & Answers are hosted on
**https://expertconsult.inkling.com/store/book/
sarris-clinical-naturopathy-case-files-1**

BIBLIOGRAPHY

Fjerbaek A, Knudsen UB. Endometriosis, dysmenorrhea and diet – what is the evidence? *Eur J Obstet Gynecol Reprod Biol.* 2007;132(2):140-147.

Hansen S, Knudsen U. Endometriosis, dysmenorrhoea and diet. *Eur J Obstet Gynecol Reprod Biol.* 2013;169(2):162-171.

Hudson T. *Women's Encyclopedia of Natural Medicine.* New York: McGraw-Hill; 2008.

Trickey R. *Women, Hormones and the Menstrual Cycle: Herbal and Medical Solutions from Adolescence to Menopause.* Melbourne: Melbourne Holistic Health Group; 2012.

Wardle J. Endometriosis. In: Sarris J, Wardle J, eds. *Clinical Naturopathy: An Evidence-based Guide to Practice.* Sydney: Churchill Livingstone; 2014.

Weiss G, Goldsmith LT, Taylor RN, et al. Inflammation in reproductive disorders. *Reprod Sci.* 2009;16(2):216-229.

24 | Fibroids

Susan Arentz

PRESENTATION

A 45-year-old woman presents with **heavy menstrual bleeding** and **recurrent respiratory infections**. Her menstrual cycle is regular, with menstruation occurring every 28 days; however, three of the previous six cycles have been shorter at 23–25 days. **Two uterine fibroids** were observed on ultrasound 12 months ago—the first at 0.5 × 0.7 × 0.3 anterior intramural and the second at 0.9 × 0.7 × 1.2 posterior submucosal; these fibroids were discovered during investigations for causes of infertility. The woman and her partner have been **hoping to conceive** during the previous 5 years. The heavy bleeding (daily use of 10–12 tampons and maternity pads) started 6 months ago. During the previous 6 months she had three respiratory infections. **Three courses of antibiotics were taken** and eventually oral corticosteroids were used to resolve persistent sinusitis (she continues to take 10 mg prednisolone). **She has a busy lifestyle**, with full-time work and pressured deadlines. Her diet is generally good; however, she only consumes red meat twice per month.

Diagnostic considerations

Fibroids may contribute to heavy menstrual bleeding by increasing the myometrial surface area and endometrial volume. Normal menstrual blood loss is approximately 30 mL over 3–5 days. Blood loss of more than 7 days and 80 mL is considered elevated. The fibroids could be assessed following referral to a medical practitioner and ultrasound investigation. In the meantime the menstrual pattern, coupled with limited dietary intake of red meat (bioavailable iron), suggests this patient is at risk of iron-deficiency anaemia. Clinical signs supporting the diagnosis include the pale conjunctiva, poor venous return and cold hands and feet. Other clinical signs (not apparent in this case) include fatigue and breathlessness. A full blood count (requested by a medical practitioner) and/or iron studies would confirm the diagnosis. Iron-deficiency anaemia may complicate healthy immune function with symptomatic recurrent colds and infections.

A recent pregnancy could be another option, with the bleeding due to pregnancy loss. This could be discussed with reference to the patient's observations of other signs and symptoms and previous investigations. Other factors of interest include the patient's history of atopy, inflamed mucous membranes (respiratory and uterine), underlying mental health issues (mild anxiety due to infertility, anticipation about surgery and stressful job) and frequency of swimming during the winter months (including exposure to the cold and chlorine and potential allergy and upper respiratory tract dysbiosis).

MEDICAL CONDITIONS THAT MAY MIMIC OR AGGRAVATE FIBROID SYMPTOMS

- Pregnancy loss
- Cervical polyps
- Hypothyroidism
- Endometrial hyperplasia
- Endometrial cancer
- Adenomyosis
- Sexually transmitted infections

Treatment protocol

- The primary treatment goal is to reduce the heavy menstrual bleeding and boost immunity. Secondary treatment aims are to improve red blood cell count, reduce inflammation and improve quality of life (reduce anxiety).

- Due to this woman's interest in cooking, focus is drawn to dietary solutions. Recommendations are to increase dietary intake of red meat to four or five times per week. Other food sources of iron are identified (beans, legumes). Liver is presented as a good source of iron as well as vitamin A (it is a synergistic nutrient for healthy stomach function and iron absorption as well as essential for the health of mucous membranes (respiratory)). Phytate-containing vegetables are to be avoided in conjunction with red meat and instead accompanying foods containing ascorbic acid are emphasised to enhance iron absorption (tomatoes, avocado, etc.). Horseradish and mustards will clear mucus in the respiratory tract. Other dietary components include turmeric, ginger and garlic. Discuss recipe ideas and highlight foods with specific nutrients and therapeutic effects.

- Nutritional supplementation focuses on iron with B12 and folic acid to treat anaemia, as well as ascorbic acid with bioflavonoids for as cofactors and a tablet containing vitamin A and zinc to improve immunity and mucous membrane health.

- The herbal formula aims to improve immunity, reduce heavy menstrual bleeding, enhance digestive absorption of nutrients, improve mucous membrane tone and support mental health. Specific herbs include *Withania somnifera*, which is used to increase the Th1 immune response and improve resistance to infections and reduce allergic inflammation and anxiety. *Schisandra chinensis* will enhance liver detoxification and reduce chronic inflammation, boost immunity and improve mood. To support healthy liver metabolism of oestrogen, *Zingiber officinale* is used to increase circulation to the stomach, digestion of proteins and nutrients (including iron), regulate digestive pH and improve digestive microflora; *Panax notoginseng* is used as a uterine astringent to prevent heavy menstrual blood loss and improve endothelial (blood vessel) tone; and *Glycyrrhiza glabra* is prescribed as an anti-inflammatory with high iron content and to improve the taste of the formula (and therefore compliance).

PRESCRIPTION
Herbal formula (100 mL)

Withania somnifera 2:1	30 mL
Tienchi notoginseng 1:2	30 mL
Schisandra chinensis 1:2	25 mL
Glycyrrhiza glabra 1:1	10 mL
Zingiber officinale 1:2	5 mL
Dose: 6 mL 3 × daily	

Nutritional prescription

Iron, B12 and folic acid supplement (iron 30 mg, B12 100 mcg, folic acid 95 mcg)

Vitamin C (ascorbic acid): 940 mg with bioflavonoids (quercetin, rutin and citrus bioflavonoids (170 mg)

Vitamin A and zinc combination (zinc amino acid chelate 25 mg elemental with vitamin A 750 mcg RE, 2500 IU; vitamin B6 (pyridoxine) 50 mg; magnesium 25 mg and manganese 2 mg)

Expected outcomes and follow-up protocol

The patient is advised to keep a record of her menstrual cycle length to monitor progress. Using digital tracking with a mobile phone app is potentially more convenient than handwritten charts. Additional observations entered on to the digital tracking device can include the number of pads and tampons used during menstruation, pre- and post-menstrual symptoms, sleep quality, morning energy and respiration condition (e.g. inflammation—yes or no).

Ideally the patient will report slightly less blood flow during her first subsequent menstrual period. Dysmenorrhoea and sleep quality are intended to be improved (with no ibuprofen being taken) and no post-menstrual headache. If there is no change in morning energy and the menstrual cycle, then the herbal formula can be adjusted with increased proportions of *Panax notoginseng* and *Schisandra chinensis* (increased by 10 mL/200 mL) and reductions of licorice and *Withania somnifera* (reduced by 10 mL). Menstrual cycle improvements are expected to be observed following a minimum of 3 months' treatment; however, an initial 'trend' towards improvement should be noted, otherwise other options should be considered. In this case other additions could be *Vitex agnus-castus* and *Shatavari racemosus* and *Actaea/Cimicifuga racemosa*. Dietary intake of iron and compliance with supplements could ideally be reviewed at 4 weeks. A referral to a medical provider could be provided for further investigation of iron status and to check ongoing use of corticosteroids.

Clinical pearls

- Recurrent respiratory infections may be secondary to iron-deficiency anaemia.

- Abnormal menstrual bleeding might be secondary to endometrial cancer, and medical assessment is an important inclusion in managing women with fibroids.

- Ultimately the best treatment in this case may be surgery; however, the patient can benefit from support to reduce anxiety prior to hospital admission.

- Menstrual cycle improvements may take up to 3 months to respond; however, a trend should be observed after a month of treatment.

Expert | CONSULT

Clinical Comprehension Questions & Answers are hosted on
**https://expertconsult.inkling.com/store/book/
sarris-clinical-naturopathy-case-files-1**

BIBLIOGRAPHY

Ansari T, Ikram N, Najam-ul-Haq M, et al. Essential trace metal (zinc, manganese, copper and iron) levels in plants of medicinal importance. *J Biol Sci.* 2004;4(2):95-99.

Greenlee H, Atkinson C, Stanczyk FZ, et al. A pilot and feasibility study on the effects of naturopathic botanical and dietary interventions on sex steroid hormone metabolism in premenopausal women. *Cancer Epidemiol Biomarkers Prev.* 2007;16(8):1601-1609.

Wardle J. Dysmenorrhoea and menstrual complaints. In: Sarris J, Wardle J, eds. *Clinical Naturopathy: An Evidence-based Guide to Practice.* 2nd ed. Sydney: Churchill Livingstone; 2014.

Yang JH, Chen MJ, Chen CD, et al. Impact of submucous myoma on the severity of anemia. *Fertil Steril.* 2011;95(5):1769-1772, e1.

Yarnell E, Abascal K. Multiphasic herbal prescribing for menstruating women. *Altern Complement Ther.* 2009;15(3):126-134.

Polycystic ovarian syndrome

Jon Wardle

PRESENTATION

A 26-year-old woman presents with **irregular periods** with **heavy cramping**. She has successfully lost weight previously but has since put it back on over the past 2 years and is currently slightly **overweight**, with a BMI of 27 and a LH:FSH ratio of 2 : 1. She finds it difficult to maintain weight loss, despite eating well and exercising. She has **hair growth on her abdomen and upper lip**.

Diagnostic considerations

Irregular periods and heavy cramping can be the result of numerous hormonal issues. It is important to view other symptoms and clinical red flags as well. It is mistakenly easy to view specific conditions as having textbook levels of hormonal disturbance. In the above example, the likely polycystic ovarian syndrome (PCOS) may be viewed by many as a disorder of androgens and treatment may focus on this. However, oestrogen levels in PCOS can also be elevated and may be causative or exacerbating factors. Temperature charting offers a simple method of observing hormonal changes over the cycle, but saliva and blood tests may also be useful in determining which hormone irregularities exist. The fact that this patient is overweight should also be considered. Although a herbal formulation will help to modulate hormones, this is unlikely to be as effective as ensuring appropriate weight loss. The major factors in PCOS are being overweight and insulin resistance. While patients may be focused on their menstrual cycle and anovulation, treatment is rarely effective if these causative factors are present. The consultation should pay as much attention to exploring dietary and lifestyle factors as it does to reproductive symptoms. In any presentation where amenorrhoea exists pregnancy should be excluded first.

MEDICAL CONDITIONS THAT MAY MIMIC OR AGGRAVATE PCOS SYMPTOMS

- Response to environmental disruptions
- Hyperprolactinaemia
- Cushing's syndrome
- Thyroid disorders
- Amenorrhoea
- Ovarian tumours
- Pregnancy

Treatment protocol

- The primary treatment rationale for herbal medicine treatment is to regulate hormone feedback and production mechanisms—that is, to encourage ovulation and reduce follicle-stimulating hormone (FSH) and androgen levels.

- Zinc is used to reduce androgen conversion in relation to PCOS generally and hirsutism specifically (given there is a small body of evidence for this indication). *Mentha spicata* tea is also used for this reason.

- Her dietary recommendations focus on weight reduction and on regulating blood sugar levels. Initial protein supplementation is recommended until dietary changes become consistent. The patient is also advised to begin a higher protein diet and to reduce her refined carbohydrates. She can also be provided the names of several recipe books to help with this. Recipes to help her incorporate foods such as legumes may also be beneficial. She is also advised to increase her consumption of vegetables, particularly cruciferous, and to keep a diet diary for her next visit.

- Lifestyle factors that discourage inflammation-mediating hormonal factors are encouraged by using therapies that increase fitness, improve sleep and reduce stress.

Expected outcomes and follow-up protocols

In this case the patient is reluctant to pursue an exercise regimen due to her condition. Many patients who have PCOS research their condition extensively and are often aware of the effect of androgenic hormones. This may discourage some patients from activities that they associate with further encouraging masculine traits—this may include supplementation with protein or gym exercises (which could be viewed as encouraging masculine muscular development).

PRESCRIPTION

Herbal formula

Tablet combination:
Actaea/Cimicifuga racemosa: 300 mg dry root
Glycyrrhiza glabra: 850 mg dry root
Paeonia lactiflora: 850 mg dry root
Dose: 1 tablet 3 × daily
Mentha spicata infusion (5 g), iced or hot PRN

Nutritional prescription

Zinc amino acid chelate: 15 mg at night
Protein meal supplement

Lifestyle advice

Moderate balanced exercise: qi gong and incidental physical activity
Dietary improvement (high-protein, low-carbohydrate diet)

Educating patients will help to ensure compliance but also to alleviate patient concerns. Encouraging incidental exercise (for example, walking for 'one album' worth of music, using public transport that is a short walk from home and work) may be more effective than more vigorous exercise, not only for compliance but also to ensure weight loss is sustained.

Many patients ignore PCOS until they unsuccessfully attempt to conceive. Even once PCOS has been resolved these patients may require further preconception care on a more individual basis. Referral to a fertility program or specialist may be warranted. Insulin resistance and blood sugar management is important in PCOS—therefore naturopathic treatments (such as *Gymnema sylvestre* or chromium) may need to be considered along with a low-glycaemic-index or low-carbohydrate diet.

Treatment needs to be looked at long term. It may be months before the initial menstrual bleeding (which may seem 'excessive' in both volume and timeframe by normal standards once it does finally arrive). Patients need to be counselled on this before embarking on treatment to ensure they know what to expect and to ensure they do not get disheartened by the lack of immediate results. Charting can be a useful tool to indicate changes in hormone levels that are getting closer to those required for ovulation, even when menstrual changes are not apparent. Patients with amenorrhoea may also require a change in their prescription at the point of their first menstrual bleed to assist their cycle to become regular.

Reduction of hirsutism is also a long-term treatment. Hair follicles will often take 3–6 months (their life cycle) before effects are observed in women with PCOS. It may be prudent to counsel them to make cosmetic adjustments until then if this is a big concern, in addition to counselling them on the long timeframe of treatment. Few herbal treatments (such as *Mentha spicata*) are useful for treating hirsutism.

Clinical pearls

- Prioritise dietary and lifestyle modification first—these approaches are far more effective than any medication (natural or otherwise), and any medication is unlikely to work until these are addressed.

- Address the other risk factors that are associated with PCOS.

- Part of the role of a naturopath in weight management is to identify appropriate foods and exercises that will ensure patient compliance.

- PCOS can be an intractable condition, and PCOS treatment can be a long process. Ensure the patient is appropriately counselled about this, and engage them in their treatment for better compliance.

- Hirsutism treatment is unlikely to see results within the life cycle of current hair follicles (3–6 months). If this is an issue, temporary cosmetic removal may be required.

Expert | CONSULT

Clinical Comprehension Questions & Answers are hosted on
https://expertconsult.inkling.com/store/book/
sarris-clinical-naturopathy-case-files-1

BIBLIOGRAPHY

Giallauria F, Palomba S, Vigorito C, et al. Androgens in polycystic ovary syndrome: the role of exercise and diet. *Semin Reprod Med*. 2009;27(4):306-315.

Huang S, Chen A. Traditional Chinese medicine and infertility. *Curr Opin Obstet Gynecol*. 2008;20(3):211-215.

Hudson T. *Women's Encyclopedia of Natural Medicine*. New York: McGraw-Hill; 2008.

Kalantaridou S, Makrigiannakis A, Zoumakis E, et al. Stress and the female reproductive system. *J Reprod Immunol*. 2004;62(1-2):61-68.

Trickey R. *Women, Hormones and the Menstrual Cycle: Herbal and Medical Solutions From Adolescence to Menopause*. Melbourne: Melbourne Holistic Health Group; 2012.

Wardle J. PCOS. In: Sarris J, Wardle J, eds. *Clinical Naturopathy: An Evidence-Based Guide to Practice*. Sydney: Churchill Livingstone; 2014.

26 | General menstrual complaints

Jon Wardle

PRESENTATION

A 24-year-old woman comes into the clinic presenting with **severe menstrual cramping** each cycle. The pain is described as 'acute and stabbing'. Over time, **her periods have not become heavier but the pain is getting worse**. They are **relieved after the first few days**. She also gets **anxious** and **'moody'** before her cycle begins.

Diagnostic considerations

Although various diagnoses can often present in menstrual disorders, naturopathic treatment focuses not on treatment of particular disorders but on restoring a normal menstrual cycle. Pain reduction in dysmenorrhoea, however, is the most commonly sought treatment in those with premenstrual syndrome (PMS), even where other conditions are present (e.g. in this case anxiety and mood swings before menstruation). Many of the other symptoms of PMS are related to the same underlying issues as dysmenorrhoea, and they can be treated concurrently. A symptomatic treatment for menstrual cramping should be given in line with this request; however, returning to a normal menstrual cycle should be the focus of treatment. This can be done through a variety of mechanisms but most commonly with hormone regulation via the hypothalamic–pituitary–ovarian (HPO) axis.

While PMS is often used as an all-encompassing moniker for menstrual complaints, menstrual symptoms do not occur only prior to menstruation. Dysmenorrhoea is 'painful menstruation' and is the most common menstrual complaint, as well as having the most potential to substantially interfere with patients' lives. In fact, dysmenorrhoea is the most frequent gynaecological problem in adolescent females (the prevalence is 80–90%). Daily activities are frequently affected, and it is the most common cause of regular absenteeism in young women. Exploring the impact of PMS should therefore be an integral part of the consultation.

Primary dysmenorrhoea classically presents as a cramping lower abdominal pain that usually begins the day before menstruation. The pain gradually eases after the start of menstruation and is sometimes gone by the end of the first day of bleeding. Primary dysmenorrhoea occurs in a high percentage of young women only in ovulatory cycles, and the pain is normally limited to the first 48–72 hours of menstruation. **Secondary dysmenorrhoea** may occur during other parts of the menstrual cycle and can be either relieved or worsened by menstruation. Pain from secondary dysmenorrhoea is often described as dull and aching rather than being spasmodic or cramping in nature. It can occur before menstruation (up to 1 week) or get worse once menstruation starts.

Consultation should focus on eliciting more details about the root cause of menstrual dysfunction. Inflammation and inflammatory mediators should also be addressed, as they can worsen symptoms. PMS is highly associated with several risk factors including smoking, diet, exercise, weight (both underweight and overweight) and caffeine. Any treatment should therefore also focus on removing potentially aggravating factors. Psychological factors can be either a cause of some symptoms

IMPORTANT DIAGNOSTIC/CLINICAL CONSIDERATIONS

Fluid and electrolyte balance
- Aldosterone excess
- High sodium:potassium ratio
- Renin/angiotensin abnormalities

Hereditary factors
- Genetic risk

Hormonal factors
- Oestrogen deficiency
- Oestrogen excess
- High oestrogen:progesterone ratio
- Progesterone deficiency
- High prolactin

Inflammatory mediators
- Prostaglandin excess
- Prostaglandin deficiency

Psychological factors
- Poor coping skills
- Poor self-esteem
- Beliefs about menstrual cycle

Social factors
- Current/former sexual relationships
- Stress
- Cultural/societal attitudes about PMS
- Poor social networks

Biochemical factors
- Various vitamin and mineral deficiencies
- Dopamine deficiency

(e.g. anxiety resulting in more pronounced pain) or a clinical manifestation (e.g. due to the influence of hormone imbalances on serotonin levels). Psychological factors should be explored during the consultation.

Treatment protocol

- The patient is prescribed a herbal tablet of *Vitex agnus-castus* to help modulate HPO activity. A combination herbal tablet consisting of *Corydalis ambigua*, *Zingiber officinale* and *Viburnum opulus* is also given to provide symptomatic relief due to providing antispasmodic, anti-inflammatory and analgesic actions.

- The patient is also prescribed 6000 mg of fish oil daily to provide anti-inflammatory action and address nutritional deficiencies that become apparent from analysing her diet.

- The patient is also given dietary advice. She is told to initially avoid foods that are commonly associated with inflammatory mediators (wheat and bovine dairy) and to increase consumption of foods rich in anti-inflammatory fatty acids such as fish (tuna particularly), avocado and nuts. She should increase fibre in her diet, including the addition of legumes and whole grains. Her diet is amended to increase the variety of foods.

- Self-care methods are also advised, not only to empower the patient as a part of her own care but also because these are some of the most effective symptomatic treatments available. This includes topical application of warmth (via a hot water bottle, massage with warming liniment or a Moxa stick).

- Lifestyle factors are also addressed by designing a physical activity plan that fits within her lifestyle. Yoga may be eventually chosen in this case, which can provide the additional benefit of reducing anxiety and improving sleep.

Expected outcomes and follow-up protocols

Noticeable improvement should occur within the first cycle and continue throughout the cycles. After a few cycles of noticeably less pain the symptomatic treatments should be ceased and the prescription should focus on HPO modulation and its effectors only. It may be difficult for the patient to adhere to dietary restrictions (e.g. to completely remove dairy and wheat), so these should be monitored using a symptoms and dietary diary. In many cases, dietary improvement alone will result in improved symptoms, and in some cases symptoms may not be related to diet at all. Even where potentially aggravating foods are eaten, counselling on the importance of consuming these as part of a varied diet is beneficial. Patients should be taught to focus on less-processed versions of these foods (e.g. wholegrain wheat products and fermented or cultured dairy products).

PRESCRIPTION
Herbal formula (tablets)

Vitex agnus-castus 1 tablet daily: 1000 mg
Corydalis ambigua: 600 mg
Zingiber officinale: 400 mg
Viburnum opulus: 400 mg
1 tablet × daily

Nutritional prescription

Omega-3 fish oil capsules: 6000 mg daily

Lifestyle prescription

Moderate balanced exercise: yoga
Good sleep hygiene and mindfulness meditation
Dietary improvement including specific avoidance of potentially aggravating foods

The patient should return periodically for health visits, at which stage she may be confident and able to cease symptomatic treatments. Where treatment has been successful, symptoms can still flare up occasionally. Encouraging and educating the patient throughout treatment can empower the patient to become aware of the situations causing these flare-ups and be able to alter diet and lifestyle accordingly.

Clinical pearls

- Menstrual problems are not associated with simple hormone excess or deficiency but a complex interconnection of factors that interfere with the HPO axis.

- PMS symptoms are often treated successfully by ameliorating underlying causes with dietary and lifestyle modifications—women are not designed to experience menstrual 'dysfunction' once a month.

- Symptomatic treatment is very important. However, smooth muscle relaxants or analgesics should only be considered a temporary solution, and treating the underlying factors should be prioritised.

- Treating primary dysmenorrhoea should see positive results within the first one or two cycles. Secondary dysmenorrhoea requires treatment of its causative aetiology and is often more complex.

Expert | CONSULT

Clinical Comprehension Questions & Answers are hosted on
**https://expertconsult.inkling.com/store/book/
sarris-clinical-naturopathy-case-files-1**

BIBLIOGRAPHY

Daley A. The role of exercise in the treatment of menstrual disorders: the evidence. *Br J Gen Pract.* 2009;59(561):241-242.

Hudson T. *Women's Encyclopedia of Natural Medicine.* New York: McGraw-Hill; 2008.

Ryu A, Tae-Hee K. Premenstrual syndrome: a mini review. *Maturitas.* 2015;82(4):436-440.

Trickey R. *Women, Hormones and the Menstrual Cycle: Herbal and Medical Solutions From Adolescence to Menopause.* Melbourne: Melbourne Holistic Health Group; 2012.

Wardle J. Dysmenorrhoea. In: Sarris J, Wardle J, eds. *Clinical Naturopathy: An Evidence-Based Guide to Practice.* Sydney: Churchill Livingstone; 2014.

27 | Perimenopausal patients

Jon Wardle

PRESENTATION

A 51-year-old female presents to the clinic with **night sweats, mild hot flushing** during the day, **abdominal bloating** and **emotional swings**. Her menstrual cycle was previously 28 days with mild cramping and light flow. In the past 12 months her menstrual flow has slowly become **heavier with clotting and cramping**, and her **cycle has slowly shortened** to approximately 19–21 days. She is **irritable** and **tired**. Her **sleep is poor** because she wakes during the night due to intense sweating.

Diagnostic considerations

The menopause is a natural process that needs to be supported, not treated. Perimenopause is a natural part of the lifecycle and therefore symptoms are not necessarily indicative of pathology. Improving health parameters more generally will improve menopausal outcomes. Various lifestyle and dietary habits can have significant effects on the severity on menopausal symptoms, so treatment should focus on ensuring optimal health. Vasomotor symptoms will be experienced by over half of all perimenopausal women and are usually the symptom immediately linked with the menopause transition; vasomotor symptoms are only one symptom precipitated by the hormonal changes of the menopausal transition. Mood symptoms, urinary complaints, sleep disturbances and vaginal dryness are also commonly observed. Menopausal symptoms may have a flow-on effect into other parts of the woman's life. Insomnia, for example, may affect the physiological function of other systems and weight gain or vaginal dryness may have an impact on sexual relationships.

As naturopathic treatment of a perimenopausal patient is focused on supportive care throughout the natural menopausal transition, rather than correcting an aetiological or pathological condition, a broader clinical enquiry that extends beyond symptoms relating to oestrogen deficiency needs to be undertaken. Enquiries need to be made about mental state—anger and irritability, depression, moodiness, loss of self-esteem and sleeping difficulties. Sexual function and urinary function also need to be explored in depth. It is also important to realise that not only is the menopause a time of great hormonal change but mid-age in Western societies is also a stage of great cultural transition. The impacts of these changes (for example, children moving out, career progression, the death of parents, possible relationship ruts), particularly on the psychological factors of health, should also be explored. It should also be remembered that, as a transitional stage later in life, patients are unlikely to be as physiologically youthful as they once were. Many changes may be associated not with the menopause but with ageing itself.

Many practitioners tend to underestimate the effects of perimenopausal symptoms on their patients. However, fewer than 25% of women experience a (relatively) symptom-free menopause and more than 25% of women experience debilitating symptoms. The importance of support, empathy and education in treatment should not be ignored in patients undergoing the menopausal transition, as many women turn to practitioners for an explanation and reassurance rather than treatment. There remains a stigma in Western societies around the menopausal transition—largely due to perceived cultural links between femininity and fertility. Patients should be encouraged to explore their sexual and feminine selves and be reassured that these aspects of themselves do not diminish with the cessation of menses.

SYMPTOMS THAT MAY MIMIC MENOPAUSAL SYMPTOMS

- Other sources of hot flushes (diabetes, panic attacks, hyperthyroidism)
- General gynaecological hormone imbalances (particularly in women aged under 40)
- Medication side effects
- Every woman aged over 55 will undergo the menopausal transition; differential diagnosis should instead be used for individual symptoms rather than 'menopause'

Treatment protocol

- Oestrogen modulation to address vasomotor symptoms is prescribed. In this case this consists of *Actaea/Cimicifuga racemosa* to modulate hormone levels through their various mechanisms. Phyto-oestrogenic foods are also encouraged for the oestrogen-modulating effect.

- As anxiety is associated with aggravation of perimenopausal symptoms, *Piper methysticum* is given as an anxiolytic. This is also prescribed at night to help the patient to fall asleep naturally. This is combined with educational approaches such as counselling on sleep hygiene to improve her sleep and increase energy.

- The patient also exhibits various symptoms unrelated to her menopausal transition, which is common in patients presenting for 'menopausal treatment'. To address her digestive symptoms, *Ulmus rubra* is given to encourage healthy intestinal bacterial populations, settle digestion and reduce bloating.

- The patient can be counselled about the menopausal transition and given appropriate literature regarding the changes she could expect. This will provide reassurance that she is undergoing a natural process and lessen the stigma and anxiety of the transition that is felt by many patients. This also encourages a more active approach to addressing menopausal symptoms, which itself has been associated with better clinical outcomes.

PRESCRIPTION
Herbal formula

Actaea/Cimicifuga racemosa: 42 mg dry root
1 tablet 2 × daily
Piper methysticum: aqueous extract containing 60 mg kavalactones
2 tablets 2 × daily
Ulmus rubra: 1 tbsp bark powder at night

Lifestyle prescription

Moderate balanced exercise: yoga, tai chi
Good sleep hygiene and mindfulness meditation
Dietary improvement including specific increases of phyto-oestrogen-rich foods
Counselling and literature provided on changes she could expect during transition

Expected outcomes and follow-up protocols

Perimenopause is a natural part of the lifecycle and therefore symptoms are not necessarily indicative of pathology. The changes will result in symptoms that can be expected to continue for some time (1 year or more). Naturopathic treatment effects may not be instantaneous; for example, *Actaea/Cimicifuga racemosa* treatment may require 2 weeks to take effect and 3 months before optimal benefit can be observed. Patients should be moved towards a general health program as soon as possible to ultimately improve their symptoms and lessen their duration. If *Actaea/Cimicifuga racemosa* is not effective, adrenal tonics may be a treatment of choice to support women through the process (e.g. *Panax ginseng* or *Eleutherococcus senticosus*).

Women undergoing the menopause transition turn to complementary medicines not only to seek effective treatment but also to gain greater control over their symptoms. It is therefore essential that a strong participatory relationship is encouraged during treatment and that the naturopath does not fall into the habit of product prescribing only. Moreover, by definition the menopausal transition occurs at an age when other comorbidities are likely. These comorbidities often have a complex interrelationship with the hormonal changes observed during the menopausal transition. Mental health, sexual health and physical health of patients presenting with menopausal symptoms needs to be examined at each visit because the consistency of symptoms observed prior to the menopausal transition may no longer be current.

It should also be noted that the protective effects of female sex hormones on cardiovascular risks will also be reduced during and after the menopausal transition, with postmenopausal women having a similar cardiovascular risk profile as men. For this reason attention needs to be paid to the long-term consequences of the menopausal transition in addition to short-term symptomatic treatment. Dietary and lifestyle modification towards a healthier regimen should be considered an essential part of any menopausal consultation.

Clinical pearls

- Menopause is a natural process through which the patient needs to be supported, not treated.

- Improving health parameters more broadly will improve symptoms.

- Menopause is experienced differently by every woman; what works in many of your patients won't necessarily translate to all patients. Particular care needs to be undertaken when prescribing herbal or nutritional supplements.

- Much of the distress regarding menopause is associated with the stigma or confusion around this condition. Remind patients that this is not 'the end' of anything and provide reassurance.

- Involve patients in the treatment process, encouraging a shift to self-care modalities. This will improve symptomatic relief.

Expert | CONSULT

Clinical Comprehension Questions & Answers are hosted on
**https://expertconsult.inkling.com/store/book/
sarris-clinical-naturopathy-case-files-1**

BIBLIOGRAPHY

Coon J, Pittler MH, Ernst E. Trifolium pratense isoflavones in the treatment of menopausal hot flushes: a systematic review and meta-analysis. *Phytomedicine*. 2007;14(2-3):153-159.

Hudson T. *Women's Encyclopedia of Natural Medicine*. New York: McGraw-Hill; 2008.

Leach M, Moore V. Black cohosh (*Cimicifuga* spp.) for menopausal symptoms. *Cochrane Database Syst Rev*. 2012;(9):CD007244.

Trickey R. *Women, Hormones and the Menstrual Cycle: Herbal and Medical Solutions From Adolescence to Menopause*. Melbourne: Melbourne Holistic Health Group; 2012.

Wardle J. Menopause. In: Sarris J and Wardle J. *Clinical Naturopathy: An Evidence-Based Guide to Practice*. Sydney: Churchill Livingstone; 2014.

28 | Assisted reproduction (IVF)

Karen Martin

PRESENTATION

A 38-year-old female presents for **naturopathic support during in vitro fertilisation (IVF)**. She has one child aged 15 years conceived naturally. She has had a change in life circumstances and has decided she would like to have another child. She has a **history of endometriosis**. Her **body mass index is 29.2** and she is **very prone to stress and anxiety**. Neither she nor her partner are cigarette smokers, they generally consume only moderate amounts alcohol, and she has a moderate caffeine intake of approximately three cups of coffee daily. She is currently taking a preconception multivitamin. She **conceived naturally 9 months ago**; however, the **pregnancy was ectopic** and resulted in **loss of fallopian tube**. In the past 8 months she has undergone **three attempts at IVF, all of which were unsuccessful**. Her fourth IVF procedure is scheduled in 6 weeks' time. She has decided that if this attempt at IVF is not successful she will not persist with assisted reproductive technology (ART) due to a combination of stress and financial constraints. Her reason for presenting to the clinic is so that if she is not successful she can discontinue treatment feeling that she 'has done everything she could'.

Diagnostic considerations

Naturopathic support for IVF and/or treatment for subfertility should, wherever possible, involve both partners. Approximately 30% of infertility or subfertility problems originate in the female partner, 30% in the male partner, 30% as a result of issues in both, and approximately 10% remain unexplained. Advancing maternal age contributes heavily to subfertility and infertility, and this risk factor is non-modifiable. Women experience a natural decline in fertility and by the time they are aged in their late 30s their fertility is expected to be substantially reduced compared with when they were in their early 20s. Being overweight or obese is a

131

modifiable risk factor for subfertility in both males and females, although sudden weight loss is to be avoided because this may also adversely affect fertility. Stress and anxiety is a contributing factor to subfertility and is also one of the major reasons cited for discontinuing ART. Subfertility in couples may contribute to relationship problems, which may further exacerbate stress and anxiety. Other stressors may also be present such as financial concerns (possibly exacerbated by the cost of ART), as well as general life difficulties.

CONDITIONS/MEDICATIONS THAT MAY BE ASSOCIATED WITH SUBFERTILITY

- Polycystic ovarian syndrome
- Endometriosis
- Fibroids
- Diminished ovarian reserve
- Autoimmune disease
- Thyroid disorders
- Low sperm quality
- Steroid–hormone imbalance
- Obesity (male or female)
- Some prescription medications
- Recreational drugs

Treatment protocol

- Dietary advice to moderate weight loss using nutrient-dense foods is very important with overweight patients presenting for IVF/ART support. The diet should be rich in whole plant-based foods and omega-3 fatty acids, and low in overly processed and animal-based foods.
- Caffeine should be reduced to less than 200 mg daily.
- Discontinuing alcohol will assist fertility and aid weight loss.
- Stress management is important. Referral to a qualified counsellor experienced with IVF should be a priority for patients presenting with high stress and/or anxiety.
- Adjuvant stress management techniques such as massage may be incorporated into the treatment plan.
- The preconception multivitamin should be continued. Any additional nutritional supplements should be prescribed based on individual patient assessment.
- Herbal medicines are not recommended during IVF cycles. If the patient is taking herbal medicines, these should be discontinued at least one week

prior to the patient beginning any conventional drugs associated with their IVF treatment.

- Acupuncture can be considered as an adjuvant therapy for all IVF patients.

PRESCRIPTION
Lifestyle prescription

Dietary guidelines and meal plans to facilitate moderate weight loss

Moderate graded exercise

Caffeine-free and low-caffeine drinks to replace coffee, tea and other caffeine-containing beverages

Stress management techniques and strategies

Appropriate preconception multivitamin

Discontinue any herbal medicines

Expected outcomes and follow-up protocols

Patients undergoing dietary change during a time of high stress may require additional support to assist them in achieving their nutritional goals. Ideally weight loss in overweight individuals should be no more than 500 g per week, as extreme weight loss may exacerbate subfertility. If the previous weight gain was the result of poor food choices then additional support may be required to maintain better choices and discourage reverting to previous habits under stress. A balance may be required between providing support without adding pressure because ART/IVF patients are often heavily weighted with conventional medical appointments and the addition of further appointments may exacerbate stress levels.

The period of highest stress with IVF patients is often the 2-week wait between embryo transfer and the first blood test to check for conception, and stress management may be required at this time. If conception has occurred, the patient should be encouraged to continue her healthy eating plan and lifestyle changes. If conception has not occurred then further treatment will vary depending on whether the patient wishes to continue trying or whether they decide to discontinue.

Clinical pearls

- Where possible, subfertility patients should be treated as a couple, with both participating in appropriate dietary and lifestyle modifications.

- Lifestyle factors such as cigarette smoking, exercise and caffeine and alcohol consumption should be addressed.

- Assisted-reproduction patients often experience stress and anxiety from several sources. Stress management is an important factor for these patients. Consider referral to a counsellor experienced in IVF and reproductive support.

- Herbal medications should be discontinued at least 1 week prior to beginning an IVF cycle.

Expert | CONSULT

Clinical Comprehension Questions & Answers are hosted on
https://expertconsult.inkling.com/store/book/
sarris-clinical-naturopathy-case-files-1

BIBLIOGRAPHY

Anderson K, Norman RJ, Middleton P. Preconception lifestyle advice for people with subfertility. *Cochrane Database Syst Rev.* 2010;4.

Atrash H, Jack BW, Johnson K. Preconception care: a 2008 update. *Curr Opin Obstet Gynecol.* 2008;20(6):581-589.

Li Z, McNally L, Hilder L, et al. *Australia's Mothers and Babies 2009. Perinatal Statistics Series.* Sydney: AIHW National Perinatal Epidemiology and Statistics Unit; 2011.

Sarris J. Anxiety. In: Sarris J, Wardle J, eds. *Clinical Naturopathy: An Evidence-Based Guide to Practice.* 2nd ed. Sydney: Elsevier; 2014.

Steel A, Martin K. Fertility, preconception care and pregnancy. In: Sarris J, Wardle J, eds. *Clinical Naturopathy: An Evidence-Based Guide to Practice.* 2nd ed. Sydney: Elsevier; 2014.

29 | Subfertility

Amie Steel

PRESENTATION

A 35-year-old female presents to the clinic saying she wants to fall pregnant. She was diagnosed with **polycystic ovarian disease** 5 months ago and unintentionally became pregnant 1 week later. She **miscarried** the pregnancy at 5 weeks. She and her partner have since been actively trying to conceive for 2–3 months. Her **body mass index is 28.4** and her **umbilical:hip ratio is 0.8**. Her **menstrual cycle is irregular** and can vary between 26- and 47-day cycles. She also experiences **breast tenderness** and **depression premenstrually**. Her **libido has been diminished**, and she has not menstruated since the miscarriage. She is feeling **quite anxious** about conceiving and is waking up to five times a night.

Diagnostic considerations

The initial treatment for this case should focus on improving natural fertility via supporting her nervous system and reproductive hormones while further exploring her glucose tolerance. The effect of her polycystic ovarian disease on potential fertility and capacity to carry to term needs to be acknowledged. Hyperinsulinaemia or hyperglycaemia may promote issues in pregnancy, so these also need to be addressed as a priority for ensuring natural fertility. Prior to more aggressive treatment of her insulin sensitivity, a glucose-insulin tolerance test (GITT) needs to be ordered. Although women often present for fertility sessions alone, infertility or subfertility is rarely due to factors related to the woman alone (and in 30% of couples it is factors related to the male alone). For this reason it is recommended that her partner come for the next consultation.

Risk factors that can lower fertility need to be explored and addressed. A range of dietary constituents have been linked with various aspects of infertility including intake of *trans*-fatty acids, protein, high carbohydrates, iron, antioxidants, selenium and zinc. Psychological stress and depression is an added risk factor for reduced fertility in both females and males. Both maternal and paternal age have a bearing on the fertility level of a couple.

Another general risk factor to consider when approaching preconception care is the presence of underlying disease. Women with a chronic disease such as diabetes have an increased risk of congenital abnormalities in their offspring but are known to have improved birth outcomes when they plan their pregnancies and use preconception care.

Other conditions may affect fertility but, rather than the disease being detrimental, it is the medication used to manage the condition that is usually problematic. Several different types of medications, including hormones, antibiotics, antidepressants, pain-relieving agents and aspirin/ibuprofen when taken in the middle of the cycle, have been reported to affect female fertility. With this in mind, it is important to address any underlying health issues, resolving them where possible, to reduce reliance on medication. Alternatively, where the condition cannot be resolved, exploring substitute medication may be necessary. For this reason, treatment of subfertility and infertility needs to focus on restoring optimal health rather than focusing on a short-term endpoint of successful pregnancy.

SUGGESTIVE SYMPTOMS AND RELATED ISSUES FOR SUBFERTILITY

- Polycystic ovary syndrome
- Elevated umbilical:hip ratio
- Premenstrual symptoms
- Irregular menstrual cycle
- History of miscarriage
- Anxiety about fertility

Treatment protocol

- Due to the effects of physiological responses to stress on the reproductive hormones, anxiolytic, sedative and antidepressant herbs such as *Matricaria recutita*, *Hypericum perforatum*, *Melissa officinalis* and *Verbena officinalis* are included in the formula.

- *Asparagus racemosus* is also included as a general nervine tonic and for its capacity to support libido and conception.

- Modifications in diet to modulate blood glucose levels are an important part of treatment. To this end she is advised to reduce her dietary carbohydrate intake, with a focus on low-glycaemic carbohydrates.

- To support these changes, it is recommended that she resume regular exercise and aim for 20–30 minutes, three or four times per week.

- Preconception multivitamins are useful to address deficiencies. Any additional nutritional supplements should be prescribed based on individual patient assessment and only used when specifically indicated.

PRESCRIPTION
Herbal formula (100 mL)

Matricaria recutita 1:2	20 mL
Hypericum perforatum 1:2	15 mL
Melissa officinalis 1:2	15 mL
Verbena officinalis 1:2	20 mL
Asparagus racemosus 1:2	30 mL
Dose: 10 mL 2 × daily	

Nutritional prescription

Pregnancy multivitamin. 1 tablet daily

Lifestyle prescription

Exercise for 20–30 minutes 3–4 × weekly
Glucose tolerance test via glucose-insulin tolerance test (GITT)

Expected outcomes and follow-up protocols

Following this treatment, the next intended step would focus on more specific treatment of glucose metabolism, depending on the outcomes of the GITT. Depending upon the regularity of her menstrual cycle, *Vitex agnus-castus* could also be incorporated into her treatment plan. In this case, if she is already pregnant at her return consultation, her liquid herbal formula can be replaced with infusions of *Matricaria recutita* three times daily because 'fertility herbs' (and many other herbs) should be discontinued at this time. She should be counselled to focus on maintaining a positive mindset.

The journey to conception for couples having difficulty can be quite tumultuous and unpredictable. It is important to have a plan in mind and encourage couples to allow sufficient time for good foundations to be laid before conceiving. However, this also needs to be tempered with the often-present impatience expressed by couples who have 'tried everything' prior to their first naturopathic consultation. Furthermore, naturopaths also need to be flexible with their treatment plan and be prepared to cancel intended treatment protocols and compromise certain stages in preconception care if this does not fit in with the timeline of the couple, or alternatively if the couple unexpectedly fall pregnant outside of the intended plan. Either way, it is important that the naturopath value and appreciate the powerful role counselling and dietary and lifestyle changes can have on conception and pregnancy outcomes, rather than placing all of their focus on supplements and other such interventions.

Clinical pearls

- Women should be reassured that pregnancy is a normal part of life and normal activities should be continued where possible.

- Infertility or subfertility is rarely just a female issue. A coordinated approach involving both partners is necessary.

- There is no 'one-size-fits all' approach to preconception or pregnancy care, and an individualised approach is required.

- The treatment goal is restoring good health as often as it is treating infertility—in most cases a healthy body is a fertile body. Do not provide medications unless they are specifically indicated.

Expert | CONSULT

Clinical Comprehension Questions & Answers are hosted on
**https://expertconsult.inkling.com/store/book/
sarris-clinical-naturopathy-case-files-1**

BIBLIOGRAPHY

Anderson K, Norman RJ, Middleton P. Preconception lifestyle advice for people with subfertility. *Cochrane Database Syst Rev.* 2010;(4):CD008189.

Atrash H, Jack BW, Johnson K. Preconception care: a 2008 update. *Curr Opin Obstet Gynecol.* 2008;20(6):581-589.

Li Z, McNally L, Hilder L, et al. *Australia's Mothers and Babies 2009. Perinatal Statistics Series.* Sydney: AIHW National Perinatal Epidemiology and Statistics Unit; 2011.

Sarris J. Anxiety. In: Sarris J, Wardle J, eds. *Clinical Naturopathy: An Evidence-Based Guide to Practice.* 2nd ed. Sydney: Elsevier; 2014.

Steel A, Martin K. Fertility, preconception care and pregnancy. In: Sarris J, Wardle J, eds. *Clinical Naturopathy: An Evidence-Based Guide to Practice.* 2nd ed. Sydney: Elsevier; 2014.

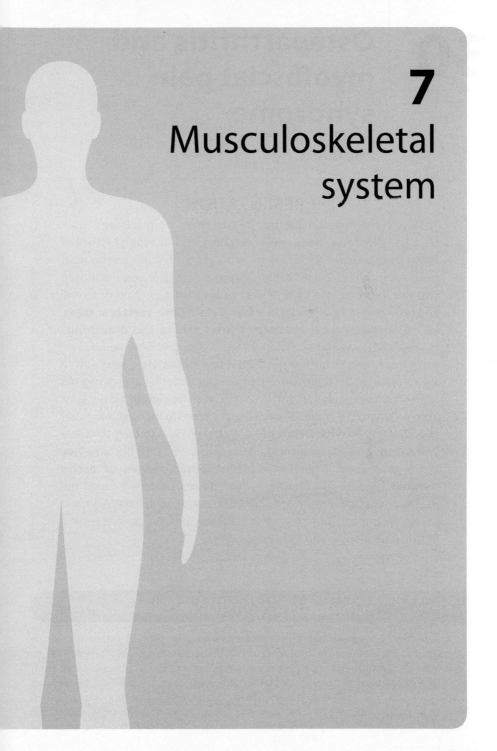

7

Musculoskeletal system

30 | Osteoarthritis and myofascial pain syndrome

Paul Orrock

PRESENTATION

A 58-year-old male builder has had to retire from full-time work because of his **lower back and knee pains**. He has a **long history of lower back pain**, which was acute in his 20s (with sciatica in his right calf) and is now recurrent depending on activity. He was diagnosed two decades ago as a **L4/5 IV disc bulge**, but now pain is central and **referring only to the local left and right para-vertebral areas**. He experiences concurrent bilateral **knee aching and 'crunching'**. His left knee was injured skiing 20 years ago, and now he finds he **can't bear weight for longer than a few hours**. He is very stiff in the morning and requires up to half an hour to get his legs going. His right shoulder is also stiff and 'crunches', and he cannot lift his arms above his head anymore. He experiences aches in his neck and other shoulder and feels he cannot put any effort in; it only feels tolerable when resting. He has previously been diagnosed with fibromyalgia.

On examination, he has multiple **limited ranges of active motions** because of pain and **trigger points** bilaterally in his trapezius, suboccipital myofascia, lumbar paravertebrals, buttocks and calves. Multiplane joint restrictions are revealed on passive testing in the lumbar spine and left knee.

Diagnostic considerations

As a first step, it is important to uncover the source of pain. A systematic physical examination is useful for exploring the somatic tissues that are tender and to reproduce the familiar pains on provocation. Important clinical insights come from palpating anatomical features to ascertain subjective pain thresholds, confirming tissue resilience and exploring trigger points. Active motion testing is required to observe a patient's pain behaviour and the provocation of pain from contractile tissues (muscles), whereas passive motion testing contrasts with active tests and provokes the non-contractile tissues (ligament/connective tissue). Special tests to stress specific features (e.g. knee meniscus, shoulder rotator cuff) are also required, as is neurological assessment in order to rule in or out nerve compression and referred/ radiating pain. Assessment of fibromyalgia scores using the widespread pain index (WPI) and somatic symptom (SS) tally is important.

The differentiation between local and/or systemic causes of somatic pain is vital for the patient's long-term outcomes. Strategies to employ include diagnostic imaging (plain x-rays of affected joints), magnetic resonance imaging if indicated (to visualise soft tissues) and laboratory tests (rheumatoid factor, erythrocyte sedimentation rate, antinuclear antibodies, C-reactive protein, full blood count to rule out infection and anaemia of chronic disease and serum uric acid to eliminate gout).

Patients with chronic diseases such as osteoarthritis have a higher rate of depression and anxiety than the general population. Osteoarthritis also has a feature of chronic pain, which can result in feelings of lowered self-worth, anxiety and depression. The practitioner needs to be aware of the effect these psychosocial aspects have on the condition and its progression, and then to educate the patient about how their psychological status can amplify pain signals. Osteoarthritis can also affect relationships and community and social activities, which are all addressed in the naturopathic assessment of the individual.

MEDICAL CONDITIONS THAT MAY PRESENT AS MYOFASCIAL PAIN

- Myofascial pain syndrome
- Fibromyalgia
- Osteoarthritis
- Bursitis
- Gout
- Calcium pyrophosphate deposition disease (CPPD/pseudogout)
- Rheumatoid arthritis

Treatment protocol

- The herbal prescription is designed for anti-inflammatory, analgesic and circulatory stimulatory actions. This may necessitate multiple treatments (e.g. a liquid tincture and a herbal tablet).

- The nutritional supplements are prescribed to focus on reducing joint pain, enhancing mobility, cartilage protection and structural modification via anti-inflammatory activity.

- Check the patient's vitamin D status. Patients with deficiency have been found to have increased incidence of musculoskeletal pain and osteoarthritis.

- The physical medicine approach aims to: stimulate circulation and drainage of muscles and joints; promote healing of tissues, enabling the exercise program to progress; enhance range of motion to optimise activities of daily living; and modify myofascial trigger points.
- Self-care modalities are encouraged to allow greater continuity of care but also to engage the practitioner in their treatment.

PRESCRIPTION
Herbal formula (100 mL)

Salix alba 1:1	25 mL
Harpagophytum procumbens 2:1	35 mL
Uncaria guianensis 1:2	30 mL
Zingiber officinale 1:2	10 mL

Dose: 5 mL 3 × daily before food

Boswellia serrata tablets: 4 g 2 × daily with food

Curcuma longa (equiv. 400 mg standardised curcumin) capsules: 3 × daily with food

Nutritional prescription

Glucosamine sulfate: 500 mg 3 × daily

Methylsulfonylmethane powder (MSM): 3 g powder 2 × daily

Vitamin D: 1000 IU/day

Physical medicine

Therapeutic massage with ginger oil once a week for 1 month, including range of motion and then maintenance—consider referral to a manual medicine practitioner

Symptomatic cold packs on affected regions

Acupuncture/pressure and/or spray and stretch for trigger points

Lifestyle prescription

Moderate strengthening exercise

Dietary adjustment to keep weight under control

Education and reassurance about managing pain—consider referral to a pain clinic

Expected outcomes and follow-up protocols

When patients present with chronic pain it is important to assess the effect this pain has on the individual's activities of daily living and their psychological wellbeing. After all, pain is described as an 'unpleasant sensory and emotional experience associated with actual or potential tissue damage, or described in terms of such damage', and because of this subjectivity, goals of management should be patient-centred. A careful recording of this functional disability on initial consultation will greatly assist when reviewing outcomes for each individual.

An important aspect of integrative medicine is how the practitioner deals with the patient taking both pharmaceutical and naturopathic medicines—the interactions and side effects, the need for immediate pain relief and the negative effect of chronic pain on mental health. For this reason, an open mind and solid knowledge of the mainstream management of pain is vital in naturopathic practice.

Musculoskeletal pain has broad systemic effects when it is limiting exercise and disturbing sleep, not the least of which are cardiovascular and metabolic consequences. Treat these patients with a holistic understanding and coach them back into optimal activity, allowing the secondary effects to self-heal. The manual therapy can be applied regularly so a therapeutic relationship is built, and motivation for lifestyle change should be included in each consult. Management in chronic degenerative conditions will mean maintenance appointments will need to be scheduled, but once a patient is adherent to the lifestyle changes and understands their condition, gradual improvement is likely over a 6-month period.

Clinical pearls

- Diagnosis is important in chronic musculoskeletal pain syndromes, as the aetiology varies from common low-grade to life-threatening.

- Chronic pain, no matter what the cause, can become centralised in the brain and alter the way a patient perceives pain in general.

- Depression is a potential consequence of chronic pain.

- Aim to optimise function and prevent worsening in chronic degenerative conditions.

- Be aware of the need for multidisciplinary care.

Expert | CONSULT

Clinical Comprehension Questions & Answers are hosted on
https://expertconsult.inkling.com/store/book/
sarris-clinical-naturopathy-case-files-1

BIBLIOGRAPHY

Axelrod L. Fibromyalgia. In: Sarris J, Wardle J, eds. *Clinical Naturopathy: An Evidence-Based Guide to Practice*. 2nd ed. Sydney: Elsevier; 2014.
Kelly A. Managing osteoarthritis pain. *Nursing*. 2006;36(11):20-21.
Merskey H, Bogduk N, eds. *Part III: Pain Terms, Classification of Chronic Pain*. 2nd ed. Seattle: IASP Task Force on Taxonomy, IASP Press; 1994.

Orrock P. Osteoarthritis. In: Sarris J, Wardle J, eds. *Clinical Naturopathy: An Evidence-Based Guide to Practice*. 2nd ed. Sydney: Elsevier; 2014.

Rosemann T, Gensichen J, Sauer N, et al. The impact of concomitant depression on quality of life and health service utilisation in patients with osteoarthritis. *Rheumatol Int*. 2007;27(9):859-863.

Wolfe F. How to use the new American College of Rheumatology fibromyalgia diagnostic criteria. *Arthritis Care Res*. 2011;63(7):1073-1074.

31 Rheumatoid arthritis

Neville Hartley

PRESENTATION

A 32-year-old Caucasian female presents with **pain, stiffness and swelling in many joints of her hands and feet**. She mentions her **sleep has been poor** for the past 2 months and that she suffers from **fatigue** on a daily basis. On further questioning she says that she is **stressed (8/10)** working full-time as a medical receptionist in a busy medical practice and looking after two young children aged 5 and 6 years. Her GP has prescribed a standard dose of ibuprofen for her arthralgia and referred her to a rheumatologist, who diagnosed **rheumatoid arthritis** after finding a **high positive rheumatoid factor** and **abnormal erythrocyte sedimentation rate**. Her diet consists of a high percentage of refined and processed foods and low fruit and vegetable intake. She attends a yoga class once a fortnight but is otherwise sedentary.

Diagnostic considerations

Treatment of the above case should include reducing the inflammatory burden placed on the joints, in addition to improving energy levels and alleviating stressors. Diagnostically, x-rays should be performed to rule out osteoarthritis, which can coexist with rheumatoid arthritis (RA) and will require different treatment interventions. In this case, a treatment approach that reduces inflammation by down-regulating the inflammatory cascade and balancing cytokine biology is indicated.

The underlying inflammatory disease activity coupled with pain and psychological distress could be the reason for her sleep disturbances and subsequent fatigue. Poor sleep and pain is a vicious cycle where pain causes sleep disturbance and poor sleep increase pain severity. In this case, a two-tiered treatment approach to reduce pain and improve sleep is recommended.

Her fatigue is a common manifestation of RA and is compounded by her poor sleep, pain, stress and dietary imbalances. Correction of the above factors should prove beneficial; however, a referral to a GP for pathology tests may be required to ascertain other causes of her fatigue. Iron studies will differentiate between iron-deficiency anaemia and anaemia of inflammation, with the latter presenting with low iron levels yet normal levels of ferritin. Her psychological stress will be contributing to the inflammation in the immune system and may worsen disease activity. Referral to a counsellor to help her work through any distress about her disease and other life stress is recommended.

MEDICAL CONDITIONS, ENVIRONMENTAL, DIETARY AND OTHER FACTORS THAT MAY MIMIC OR AGGRAVATE RA SYMPTOMS

- Systemic lupus erythematosus
- Osteoarthritis
- Gout
- Pseudogout
- Polymyalgia rheumatica
- Psychological stress
- Bacterial/virus infections
- Hypovitaminosis D
- Smoking, coffee, silica dust and pesticide exposure (may aggravate)

Treatment protocol

- The primary approach is to reduce synovial inflammation in the joints of the hands and feet. In this case, balancing cytokine biology is essential to reducing the impact of chronic inflammation and associated tissue damage. Therefore, the prescription of fish oils combined with specific herbal anti-inflammatories—curcumin (from *Curcuma longa*), *Camilla sinensis* (green tea), *Harpagophytum procumbens* and *Uncaria tomentosa*—is recommended.

- To reduce joint pain *Corydalis ambigua* and *Eschscholzia californica* have been included. A secondary clinical benefit to these herbs is a sedative and hypnotic action to improve sleep. It should also be noted that the inclusion of *Harpagophytum procumbens*, as mentioned above, would also provide analgesic activity.

- To combat stress and fatigue *Withania somnifera* and magnesium have been added. *Withania somnifera* improves energy and the ability to adapt to stress by regulating the hypothalamic–pituitary–adrenal (HPA) axis. Magnesium is a cofactor in energy production and is known to reduce stress. *Withania somnifera* also provides added anti-inflammatory action.

- Modulate the immune response via *Hemidesmus indicus*, *Uncaria tomentosa* and vitamin D supplementation. *Hemidesmus indicus* inhibits production of pro-inflammatory cytokines, and *Uncaria tomentosa* has traditionally been used to support immune function and inhibit pro-inflammatory cytokines and activation of NF-κB (a transcription factor for inflammation involved in the pathogenesis of RA). The immune-modulating potential of vitamin D has been shown to strongly correlate with significant clinical improvement in RA patients.

- Dietary modification requires correcting fatty acid profiles (reducing the omega-6 to omega-3 fatty acids ratio to 2–3:1) in order to reduce production of arachidonic acid inflammatory metabolites and the pro-inflammatory cytokines. Reducing the amount of pro-inflammatory refined and processed foods and increasing fruit and vegetable intake will improve antioxidant status. Antioxidants help suppress NF-κB and therefore reduce the production of pro-inflammatory cytokines. Adherence to a Mediterranean diet has shown benefit in RA.

- Increase physical activity by attending yoga sessions weekly and engage in low-impact aerobic conditioning such as swimming or stationary bicycling a couple of times a week. Physical activity is not only good for helping deal with stress and tension but also helps to boost the immune system. Moderate physical exercise has been shown to induce anti-inflammatory cytokines, which offers protection against inflammation and autoimmune disease. Note that, during flare-ups (active inflammatory periods), exercise should be undertaken with special care to protect the joints. Refrain from heavy resistance exercise because joint compression can increase pain and contribute to joint damage.

Expected outcomes and follow-up protocols

The diagnosis of a chronic autoimmune disease can be a stressful and disempowering experience. Consultation with a counsellor can reduce any distress the patient is experiencing. A recent study has shown that web-based interventions such as online social support and gaming increases empowerment and physical activity while decreasing medication overuse and healthcare utilisation in patients with RA.

When treating RA it is important to understand that the condition relapses and remits, therefore treatment is centred on reducing relapses (flares) and maintaining remission. Unfortunately treatment effectiveness may be difficult to determine due to spontaneous exacerbations and remissions. The patient reporting improvements when using unproven remedies may coincide with the initial stages of a spontaneous remission. Reduced joint pain and inflammation, reduced stress and fatigue and overall improvement in health is expected in the above case within 6 weeks of treatment (results may vary from individual to individual), provided there is a strict adherence to the treatment protocol. If the condition is refractory, additional interventions such as low-level laser therapy, transcutaneous electrical nerve stimulation or infrared sauna may be helpful. Failing this, the patient's rheumatologist may prescribe medications to control the disease activity. If this is the case the practitioner will have to work

PRESCRIPTION
Herbal formula (100 mL)

Withania somnifera 2 : 1	30 mL
Hemidesmus indicus 1 : 2	30 mL
Corydalis ambigua 1 : 2	20 mL
Eschscholzia californica 1 : 2	20 mL

Dose: 5 mL 3 × daily before food

Harpagophytum procumbens: equiv. 1.5 g herb
Camilla sinensis: equiv. 750 mg herb
Uncaria tomentosa: equiv. 500 mg herb
Curcuma longa: equiv. 100 mg curcumin
2 tablets 3 × daily with food

Nutritional prescription

Fish oils (EPA 300 mg, DHA 200 mg): 2 capules 2 × daily with food
Vitamin D: 1000 IU 2 caps daily with food
Magnesium amino acid chelate (75 mg elemental): 2 tablets 2 × daily after food

Lifestyle prescription

Moderate physical exercise
Good sleep hygiene and stress management strategies
Dietary improvement

in with the rheumatologist to provide support to the patient and be mindful of any herbal–nutrient–drug interactions and possible drug–nutrient depletions.

Due to the relapsing and remitting nature of RA, patients should be monitored carefully and their prescription adjusted to accommodate any changes in symptomatology and disease activity. The prescribed treatment protocol should continue until the condition has stabilised for at least 6 months and remission is evident. Eventually the herbal prescriptions can be removed, providing the patient maintains strict dietary guidelines, fish oil and vitamin D supplementation, and lifestyle advice.

Clinical pearls

- When treating RA be conscious of its relapsing and remitting nature and monitor disease activity.

- Always check for environmental triggers that may aggravate RA symptoms.

- Encourage a healthy balance between rest and activity.

- Always check stress levels.

- Always investigate dietary intake of omega-3 and omega-6 to ensure correct fatty acid profiles.

- The addition of any new medication should be investigated for side effects, possible drug–herb–nutrient interactions and drug–nutrient depletions.

Expert | CONSULT

Clinical Comprehension Questions & Answers are hosted on
https://expertconsult.inkling.com/store/book/
sarris-clinical-naturopathy-case-files-1

BIBLIOGRAPHY

Allam A, Kostova Z, Nakamoto K, et al. The effect of social support features and gamification on a web-based intervention for rheumatoid arthritis patients: randomized controlled trial. *J Med Internet Res.* 2015;17(1):e14. doi:10.2196/jmir.3510.

Hanks J, Levine D. Rheumatic conditions. In: Kauffman T, Scott R, Barr J, et al, eds. *A Comprehensive Guide to Geriatric Rehabilitation.* 3rd ed. 2014.

Hartley N, Bradbury J. Autoimmunity. In: Sarris J, Wardle J, eds. *Clinical Naturopathy: An Evidence-Based Guide to Practice.* 2nd ed. Sydney: Elsevier; 2014.

Lashley F. A review of sleep in selected immune and autoimmune disorders. *Holist Nurs Pract.* 2003;17(2):65-80.

Weiss G, Schett G. Anaemia in inflammatory rheumatic disease. *Nat Rev Rheumatol.* 2013;9:205-215.

32 Fibromyalgia

Leslie Axelrod

PRESENTATION

A 45-year-old female presents with a primary complaint of constant **generalised 'flu-like' aching pain for 2 years**, significantly worsening over the past month and affecting her ability to function. She has joint pain in her hands, shoulder and lower back region, but denies joint swelling.

She has **extreme fatigue** and **wakes five or six times per night**. In the morning she **wakes unrefreshed**. She has **difficulty with short-term memory** including retrieving words, names and what she reads. She has had a significant **increase in stress** at work recently, has a **history of a traumatic divorce** 8–9 years ago and admits to **anxiety and irritability** regarding her condition. The patient reports **chronic digestive complaints**, including bloating, indigestion, abdominal pain and carbohydrate cravings. She has a frequent history of **bladder infections treated with antibiotics**. She recently became a vegan, which improved her digestion, but not the fatigue. She has a long history of **sensitivity to chemicals**. She had a **hysterectomy** due to endometriosis and is using an oestradiol patch.

Diagnostic considerations

To exclude differential arthritic conditions, a musculoskeletal physical examination of the extremities is performed. This shows no synovitis and a normal range of movement. An examination of the tender points traditionally associated with fibromyalgia (FM) finds 12/18 above and below the waist.

Laboratory examination reveals negative or normal results for antinuclear antibodies, rheumatoid factor, cyclic citrullinated peptide (CCP), creatine kinase, aldolase, anti-RNP, thyroid, profile, cortisol, oestrogen, ferritin, methylmalonic acid and homocysteine. Significantly low levels of progesterone, testosterone and vitamin D are found. Immunoglobulin G (IgG) delayed sensitivity testing reveals multiple food sensitivities. Radiographs are unremarkable except for osteoarthritis of her first carpometacarpal joints. Brain imaging does not reveal any abnormalities.

The patient meets the 2010 FM criteria: widespread pain index (WPI > 7) and symptom severity scale (SS > 5), present for at least 3 months in the absence of another disorder that would explain the pain.

Initial treatment considerations should include improving her pain, fatigue and sleep, which are interrelated. Cognitive impairment may be attributed to the above or other aetiologies. Evaluating for other neurological conditions may be indicated. Other contributing factors include digestive, hormonal, psychological and environmental issues.

CONDITIONS THAT MAY MIMIC OR AGGRAVATE FIBROMYALGIA SYMPTOMS
- Osteoarthritis
- Rheumatoid arthritis
- Polymyositis
- Vitamin D deficiency
- Hormonal imbalance
- Myofascial pain syndrome
- Mixed connective tissue disease
- Hypothyroidism
- Food sensitivity
- Somatic disorder

Treatment protocol

- The primary approach is to improve pain and sleep. Intravenous nutritional therapies, including magnesium, calcium, B vitamins and ascorbic acid, are used to improve tender points, pain, depression and quality of life. Supplementation of 5-HTP increases the effect of serotonergic pathways, resulting in reduction of pain, insomnia and anxiety.

- Dysfunction begins at the cellular, nutritional and circulatory levels, ultimately affecting tissues and systems. D-ribose and coenzyme Q10 benefit cellular adenosine triphosphate (ATP) production. Acupuncture, manual therapy and hydrotherapy will improve tissue oxygenation and blood flow, resulting in less pain and fewer FM tender points. Aerobic exercise has been shown to be the most effective for FM. Nutritional deficiencies can result from abnormal nutrient utilisation and gastrointestinal disturbances. Magnesium and vitamin D deficiency is associated with fatigue, depression and non-specific muscle pain. Whole-body hyperthermia has been shown to increase blood flow, oxygenation and ATP release.

• Gastrointestinal issues contribute to the systemic inflammation, sensory alterations and pain. Food allergy elimination may reduce dermal IgG, intestinal permeability and dysbiosis. Probiotics, fibre and glutamine can, in part, address gut immunity and abnormal flora. If there is no improvement with dietary changes and supplementation, small intestinal bacterial overgrowth (SIBO) and/or stool analysis for bacteria and parasites should be considered. Investigation of systemic infections may be warranted due to the increased incidence of certain pathogens (i.e. mycoplasma, hepatitis C) associated with FM.

• Address the psychological issues, as well as somatic complaints. There is a significant correlation between mood, sleep and pain. *Hypericum perforatum*, *Rhodiola rosea* and *Scutellaria baicalensis* can alter serotonin pathways and act as nervines. S-adenosylmethionine (SAMe) has been shown as an effective antidepressant and treatment for FM. *Eleutherococcus senticosus*, *Schisandra chinensis* and *Rhodiola rosea* have an adaptogenic effect on the hypothalamic–pituitary–adrenal (HPA) axis and stress hormones. Adaptogens for stress and mood with counselling was indicated for this patient. Other referrals may include biofeedback, mindfulness training or other cognitive therapies.

Expected outcomes and follow-up protocols

The progression of symptom amelioration is dependent on the individual and the treatment regimen. Partial relief may be seen with initial treatment of FM while continuing to improve over weeks to months. Laboratory testing for endocrine, hormonal, gastrointestinal abnormalities or chemical sensitivities can augment a multidimensional plan. In the case above, it is essential to correct the patient's sleep patterns to assist with pain reduction. Pain-relieving pharmaceuticals may need to be considered as part of the plan in severe non-responsive cases. Lifestyle changes are an integral part of the program. Exercise will improve oxygenation of the tissues, regulation of mood, sleep and other factors. Fatigue and exercise intolerance may be a challenge for the patient to initiate and follow through. In these instances a trained professional may be indicated to improve the success of the treatment program.

Any abnormalities of the digestion should also be addressed in the intermediate term to improve barrier function and absorption; however, pain reduction should be the initial focus. Dietary changes can then be the focus, with botanical and nutraceuticals intervention used adjunctively. Dysbiotic changes are common in this cohort and re-establishing normal gut flora should be promoted. Correcting the patient's nutritional deficiencies, especially vitamin D, may yield beneficial results and can be implemented. If insomnia, anxiety and fatigue continue, a salivary cortisol test may be valuable to assess aberrations in the HPA axis. FM affects patients on a profound level, and modalities such as acupuncture and mind–body techniques can provide additional assistance with the psychological component of the condition.

PRESCRIPTION
Herbal formula

Proprietary formula containing 650 mg herbal equivalent per 1 mL, key ingredients:

Eleutherococcus senticosus 1:1
Schisandra chinensis 1:3
Rhodiola rosea 1:1
Withania somnifera 2:3
Cordyceps sinensis 1:2
Ganoderma lucidum 1:2
Camellia sinensis 1:1 95% polyphenols
Curcuma longa 1:1
Dose: 3 mL 2 × daily in the morning and early evening away from food

Nutritional prescription

Vitamin D: 5000 IU
Co-Q10: 300 mg
D-ribose: 5000 mg 2 × daily
5-HTP: 50 mg nightly at bedtime

Intravenous therapy

Micronutrient IV: Once a week × 4 weeks

Diet prescription

Food allergy elimination diet

Lifestyle prescription

Re-evaluate work situation
Increase graded exercise
Counselling

Clinical pearls

- A thorough history can help detect contributory factors and assist in forming an effective therapeutic plan.

- Rule out other medical conditions. There may be other concurrent conditions, which should be corrected.

- Restful sleep is a crucial part of the healing process.

- Diet and lifestyle should always be addressed and individualised. An anti-inflammatory, hypoallergenic diet should be included with a progressive aerobic exercise program.

- A comprehensive approach that addresses body, mind and spirit is essential.

Expert|CONSULT

Clinical Comprehension Questions & Answers are hosted on
**https://expertconsult.inkling.com/store/book/
sarris-clinical-naturopathy-case-files-1**

BIBLIOGRAPHY

Axelrod L. Fibromyalgia. In: Sarris J, Wardle J, eds. *Clinical Naturopathy: An Evidence-Based Guide to Practice*. 2nd ed. Sydney: Elsevier; 2014.

Chaitow L. *Fibromyalgia Syndrome: A Practitioner's Guide to Treatment*. 3rd ed. Churchill Livingstone; 2010.

Sampalli T, Berlasso E, Fox R, et al. A controlled study of the effect of a mindfulness-based stress reduction technique in women with multiple chemical sensitivity, chronic fatigue syndrome, and fibromyalgia. *J Multidiscip Healthc*. 2009;2:53-59.

Vasquez A. Fibromyalgia. Naturopathic rheumatology and integrative inflammology, Edition 3.5, Cundinamarca, Columbia, 2014.

33 | Tension and migraine headache

Daniel Roytas

PRESENTATION

A 28-year-old male presents with a primary complaint of **stress and tension-induced headaches**, which he has suffered from for the past 18 months. The patient explains that he is **suffering from high levels of stress** due to financial and study commitments. His headaches are often brought on immediately after exertion (exercise). During a headache the patient experiences **debilitating frontal and temporal head pain** accompanied by **increased suboccipital muscle tension, photophobia** and **nausea**. These symptoms last for approximately 4 hours and are ameliorated with bed rest.

The patient also complains of persistent **fatigue** as well as **ongoing temporomandibular joint (TMJ), neck, shoulder and lower back pain**, which is not relieved with nonsteroidal anti-inflammatory drugs (NSAIDs) or massage. All previous investigations including brain imaging, blood tests and structural assessment have returned normal findings. The patient's blood pressure is 118/77 mmHg, with a resting heart rate of 65 beats per minute. The patient's **current stress levels are 9/10**. A point-of-care pathology test assessing free oxygen radical defence (FORD) and a free oxygen radicals test (FORT) identify elevated concentrations of free radicals (oxidative stress) and a low antioxidant capacity.

Diagnostic considerations

A thorough physical inspection of the head and spine as well as cardiovascular and neurological examinations should be undertaken to rule out any underlying pathology or trauma. Medical referral may be necessary to rule out other pathologies such as intracerebral haemorrhage, mass lesions or structural abnormality. Functional pathology tests may also be warranted to rule out hormonal imbalances.

Several mechanisms are likely to be contributing to the patient's tension-type headaches. Psychological stress promotes oxidative stress and reactive oxygen species (ROS) production. ROS damage and impaired mitochondrial function result in neurogenic inflammation and fatigue. Dysfunctional mitochondria negatively affect the balance of neurotransmitters, leading to hyperexcitability of brain neurons.

Oxidative stress affecting the trigeminal nerves cause central sensitisation and neurogenic inflammation through the release of substance P, calcitonin gene-related peptide, glutamate and neurokinin A. The combination of oxidative stress, central sensitisation and neurogenic inflammation are likely to contribute significantly to the patient's tension-type headaches.

The cause of pain and muscle tension associated with tension-type headaches is unknown. It is thought that tension and tenderness of pericranial myofascial tissue in response to excessive muscle contraction, ischaemia and inflammation may cause continuous nociceptive input to neurons within the spinal dorsal horn. This results in central sensitisation, decreased descending inhibition and hyperalgesia. Central sensitisation may further stimulate other spinal nerves, contributing to muscle tension and pain in the shoulders and lower back. Increased hypothalamic–pituitary–adrenal (HPA) axis activity in response to uncontrollable cognitive stress has been proposed as a potential contributing factor of tension-type headaches; however, there is currently insufficient evidence to support this theory. Nonetheless, practitioners should still consider supporting the HPA axis in patients with tension-type headaches to ameliorate the numerous negative effects associated with chronic stress.

FACTORS THAT MAY MIMIC OR AGGRAVATE MIGRAINE SYMPTOMS

- Arterial hypertension
- Physical activity
- Intracerebral haemorrhage
- Mass lesion
- Meningitis
- Glaucoma
- Trigeminal autonomic cephalgias
- Hormonal imbalance
- Postural abnormality
- Inflammation and oxidative stress
- Mitochondrial dysfunction
- Food sensitivity
- Fatigue
- Eye strain
- Neurotransmitter imbalance

Treatment protocol

- The primary approach to treating headache should focus on determining the cause of the headache (and subtype) and towards reducing the frequency of episodes and the duration and severity of symptoms. This can be achieved through supporting mitochondrial function, reducing inflammation and oxidative stress, facilitating adenosine triphosphate (ATP) production and relieving muscular tension.

- Magnesium supplementation can be considered as a primary treatment for tension headache. It is a cofactor for ATP synthase, which is responsible for producing ATP. Magnesium stimulates serotonin release and may help to balance neurotransmitter concentrations. Magnesium is also beneficial due to its inhibitory effects on platelet aggregation, inflammation, vasospasm, mast cell degradation and nitric oxide synthesis and release. Magnesium inhibits N-methyl-D-aspartate (NMDA) receptor activity and can therefore reduce neuron hyperexcitability.

- Riboflavin (B2) is an integral component for the production of ATP. B2 is the precursor for the coenzymes flavin mononucleotide (FMN) and flavin adenine dinucleotide (FAD). FMN is an essential component of complex I and II in the electron transport chain, while FAD acts as an electron donor in the citric acid cycle. Supporting energy production pathways can significantly reduce the production of ROS metabolites in the electron transport chain. Combined, these actions may in part be of benefit in treating headaches.

- Coenzyme Q10 is an integral component of ATP production, transferring electrons from complex I and II to cytochrome C within the electron transport chain. Co-Q10 also protects mitochondria from oxidative stress and supports mitochondrial inner membrane permeability.

- A thorough dietary analysis should be undertaken to identify any foods that may be contributing to headaches. There are a range of foods associated with headache (in particular with migraine headaches) that should be excluded from the diet including cheese, chocolate, wine, citrus fruit and coffee.

- Low-level laser therapy (LLLT) is a safe and effective treatment for TMJ, neck and lower back pain. Specifically, LLLT enhances cytochrome c oxidase activity in the electron transport chain, resulting in increased ATP production. LLLT antagonises ROS formation, modulates the release of inflammatory cytokines and induces smooth muscle relaxation. LLLT may also be effective for tension-type headaches by minimising chronic nociceptive input into the central nervous system.

PRESCRIPTION

Nutritional prescription

Co-Q10: 1 capsule (150 mg) 1 × daily after food
Magnesium amino acid chelate: 1 scoop (300 mg elemental) 1 × daily after food
Vitamin B2 (riboflavin): 1 tablet (100 mg) 1 × daily after food

Lifestyle prescription

Limit intense physical exercise (light walking < 30 minutes per day), increase water intake to 2 L, modify diet to include two serves of fruit and five serves of vegetables and limit tyramine-rich foods, alcohol and refined carbohydrates

Additional therapies

Low-level laser therapy (904 nm)
1–2 treatments per week for 6 weeks

Expected outcomes and follow-up protocols

A reduction in the severity, frequency and duration of headaches is expected within 2 weeks of commencing supplementation and LLLT. Relying on red blood cell magnesium assays to gauge the effect of treatment is not recommended because they tend to only be useful in individuals with a frank deficiency. Patients with tension-type headaches who benefit from magnesium are encouraged to adhere to ongoing supplementation for a prophylactic effect to be maintained. LLLT can be administered at least twice per week for the first fortnight. If pain in the neck and lower back still persists after 2–4 weeks, consider referral to a physical therapist.

Supplementation of riboflavin and co-Q10 is expected to result in a prophylactic effect within 3–6 months; however, relief may be achieved within a shorter time frame. It is imperative to schedule follow-up consultations to monitor compliance, as patients may become complacent with treatment, especially if the time between headache episodes is extended.

Dietary modification should focus on excluding foods that may be triggering headaches. Refined and processed foods should also be minimised and replaced with whole grains, fruits and vegetables. The patient should also minimise alcohol and coffee intake and consider consumption of green tea. These modifications are aimed at reducing FORT (oxidative stress) and increasing FORD (antioxidant capacity) plasma concentrations.

Patients can be made aware that the treatments outlined above are a prophylactic and not intended to provide symptomatic relief during a headache. Instructing patients to keep a 'headache diary' that details severity, frequency and duration of symptoms is recommended to gauge the efficacy of treatment over time. It is important that a referral be made for further medical investigation if the patient's symptoms become worse, or if new symptoms develop.

Clinical pearls

- Tension-type headache sufferers may excrete excessive amounts of magnesium (especially those who are stressed) and are therefore at increased risk of magnesium deficiency.

- Hypomagnesaemia frequently occurs in conjunction with other electrolyte imbalances such as hypokalaemia, hyponatraemia, hypocalcaemia and hypophosphataemia.

- It is important that a referral be made for further medical investigation if a patient with tension-type headache symptoms becomes worse, or if new symptoms such as seizure, blackouts or confusion develop.

- While long-term use of B2 is not expected to cause side effects, it is advisable to inform the patient that B2 supplementation may cause bright yellow discolouration of the urine.

Expert | CONSULT

Clinical Comprehension Questions & Answers are hosted on
https://expertconsult.inkling.com/store/book/
sarris-clinical-naturopathy-case-files-1

BIBLIOGRAPHY

Ashina S, Bendtsen T, Ashina M. Pathophysiology of migraine and tension type headache. *Reg Anesth Pain Med.* 2012;16(1):14-18.

Cottingham P. Migraine. In: Sarris J, Wardle J, eds. *Clinical Naturopathy: An Evidence-Based Guide to Practice.* 2nd ed. Sydney: Elsevier; 2014.

Gaul C, Diener H, Danesch U, et al. Improvement of migraine symptoms with a proprietary supplement containing riboflavin, magnesium and Q10: a randomized placebo controlled, double blind, multicenter trial. *J Headache Pain.* 2015;16(32):1 8.

Franco A, Goncalves D, Castanharo S, et al. Migraine is the most prevalent primary headache in individuals with tempromandibular disorder. *J Orofac Pain.* 2009;24(3):287-292.

Kato M, Kogawa E, Santos C, et al. TENS and low-level laser therapy in the management of tempromandibular disorders. *J Appl Oral Sci.* 2006;14(2):130-135.

Leistad R, Stovner L, White L, et al. Noradrenaline and cortisol changes in response to low-grade cognitive stress differ in migraine and tension type headache. *J Headache Pain.* 2007;8:157-166.

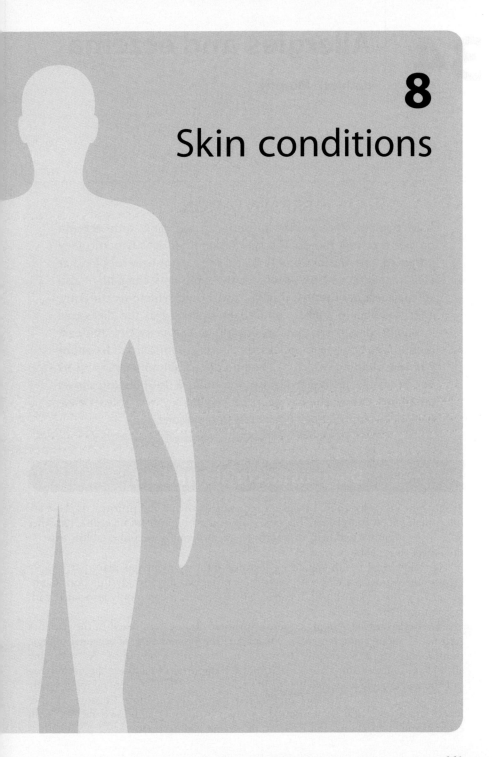

8
Skin conditions

34 Allergies and eczema

Kathleen Murphy

PRESENTATION

A 26-year-old office worker presents to the clinic with **eczema on her face and hands**. The skin around her eyes is particularly **inflamed, dry and extremely itchy**; she cannot help rubbing her eyes frequently, which exacerbates the symptoms. The patient also suffers **seasonal rhinitis**, though displays no symptoms currently, and is allergic to animal dander. She understands the diet's role in skin conditions and has cut out gluten and dairy over the past month, with nominal improvement. She also complains of **frequent gas and bloating**, which has been reduced but not eliminated by her recent change in diet. **Immunoglobulin G (IgG) testing shows an allergy to soy**; she has been consuming soy milk at least once daily since removing dairy products from her diet.

Diagnostic considerations

Treatment of this case should focus on reducing erythema and pruritus, as these are the patient's main complaints. The use of short-term topical and ingestible remedies to reduce symptoms will help to improve patient compliance and establish trust in the longer therapeutic process.

Gastrointestinal health should be factored into her treatment plan, particularly because the patient presents with symptoms of regular digestive dysfunction. Compromised gastrointestinal health, particularly dysbiosis, is commonly associated with developing atopic disease.

The overlap between atopic conditions should also be considered in the patient's treatment. Though not her main complaint, the presentation of seasonal allergic rhinitis suggests an overactive immune hypersensitivity response. As with any allergic and inflammatory skin condition, it is important to address the underlying cause(s) and exclude suspected diet or lifestyle factors. Thorough case taking is vitally important, as eczema often presents in response to one or more stressors. Further investigations may also be warranted in order to identify additional factors, both external and endogenous, contributing to eczema pathogenesis.

OTHER CONDITIONS TO CONSIDER IN THE DIFFERENTIAL DIAGNOSIS

- Psoriasis
- Candidal intertrigo
- Erythema multiforme
- Lichen planus
- Lupus erythematosus
- Dermatitis herpetiformis

Treatment protocol

- The recent diagnosis of an allergy to soy beans requires immediate elimination of foods containing this ingredient from the patient's diet. This is particularly important in light of the fact that soy products feature regularly in her diet, which has increased significantly (as a dairy substitute) over the past month. Along with this, there should be overall dietary improvement, focusing on adequate hydration and increased intake of nutrient-dense foods to help nourish the skin, reduce inflammation and modulate the immune response.

- Immune modulation should be incorporated in order to dull the hypersensitivity response. This may include use of traditional anti-allergy herbs such as *Albizia lebbeck* and nutrients such as vitamin C, B6 and zinc.

- Alterative, or depurative, herbs can help to cleanse the system and relieve inflammatory skin symptoms. Examples include *Urtica dioica, Arctium lappa, Rumex crispus* and *Centella asiatica*.

- Essential fatty acids are recommended to help nourish the skin and halt the inflammation cascade, a key feature in eczema's pathogenesis.

- To address gastrointestinal health and promote appropriate bacterial balance, probiotic supplementation may be beneficial, particularly *Lactobacillus rhamnosus*, along with additional dietary support by including fermented foods.

- Modulating stress through mindfulness practice and regular exercise may prove beneficial, along with nutrients that support nervous system function such as magnesium and adaptogenic herbs such as *Withania somnifera*.

- The role of oxidative stress should be considered because it can place further stress on the immune system and contribute to ongoing symptoms. Antioxidant nutrients such as vitamin C and zinc may be appropriate and will also modulate the immune system.

- Topical emollient treatments help to soothe inflamed and dry skin and the addition of botanicals such as *Calendula officinalis*, *Stellaria media* or *Matricaria recutita* can also provide significant relief.

PRESCRIPTION
Herbal formula (100 mL)

Echinacea spp. 1:2	20 mL
Albizia lebbeck 1:2	25 mL
Urtica dioica (leaf) 1:2	15 mL
Arctium lappa 1:2	20 mL
Centella asiatica 1:2	20 mL
Dose: 5 mL 3 × daily	

Nutritional prescription

Probiotic complex: 10^9 CFU/g—1 capsule daily with food
Omega-3 fish oil: 1000 mg—2 capsules 2 × daily with food
Zinc: 30 mg elemental—1 tablet daily with food

Lifestyle prescription

Dietary improvements, including removing known allergens
Increased water consumption
30 minutes of exercise (walking/yoga) daily and mindfulness practice

Expected outcomes and follow-up protocol

An initial follow up within 2–4 weeks is recommended to monitor any change in symptoms and assess how the patient is complying with the therapeutic recommendations. Chronic inflammatory skin conditions such as eczema often take time, sometimes months, to improve significantly, and it is important to explain this to the patient to set realistic expectations and ensure continued compliance.

Using a rating scale for level of inflammation, discomfort, itchiness etc. can help track gradual improvements and provide a reference for patients regarding the progression of their treatment. It should also be noted that acute, symptomatic relief can and should be provided as part of a treatment plan that includes short- and long-term health goals.

For some patients, symptoms may worsen for a short period of time at the outset of treatment, before beginning to improve. If this does occur, verbal reassurance and close monitoring of the patient is recommended. In cases where, after continued treatment, there is no significant improvement or an aggravation of the condition, consider referral to the patient's GP for further assessment by a dermatologist and/or allergy specialist.

Clinical pearls

- Identifying allergenic triggers is essential for successfully managing eczema and associated symptoms.

- Symptomatic treatment, including topical remedies, will help to reduce patient discomfort and improve compliance while working to identify the underlying cause.

- Support digestion and address signs of dysbiosis, such as bloating and abdominal discomfort.

Expert | CONSULT

Clinical Comprehension Questions & Answers are hosted on **https://expertconsult.inkling.com/store/book/ sarris-clinical-naturopathy-case-files-1**

BIBLIOGRAPHY

DiNicola C, Kekevian A, Chang C. Integrative medicine as adjunct therapy in the treatment of atopic dermatitis – the role of traditional Chinese medicine, dietary supplements, and other modalities. *Clin Rev Allergy Immunol.* 2013;44(3):242-253.

Ismail IH, Licciardi PV, Tang ML. Probiotic effects in allergic disease. *J Pediatr Child Health.* 2013;49(9):709-715.

Leach M. The dermatological system. In: Hechtman L, ed. *Clinical Naturopathic Medicine.* Sydney: Elsevier; 2012.

Steel A. Inflammatory skin disorders – atopic eczema and psoriasis. In: Sarris J, Wardle J, eds. *Clinical Naturopathy: An Evidence-Based Guide to Practice.* 2nd ed. Sydney: Elsevier; 2014.

35 | Acne vulgaris

Amie Steel

PRESENTATION

A 21-year-old female presents to the clinic with **inflamed acne comedones and pustules** on her cheeks and chin. Her skin has been a problem for the past 4 or 5 years, but the problem has increased in severity over the past 2 months. She is a student, and she finds **managing work and study quite stressful**. She has not noticed any connection between her acne and her menstrual cycle. She **reports a strong hunger signal** and craves both hot chips and sweet foods. This is reflected in her **diet, which contains refined carbohydrates and fried fatty foods**.

Diagnostic considerations

Prior to developing a treatment plan for a patient with acne lesions it is important to ensure other possible underlying conditions are not overlooked. Conditions that affect hormonal modulation or inflammation can result in acne. The exact sequence of the pathophysiological development of lesions is still unclear. The dominant hypothesis at this stage focuses on increased circulating androgens stimulating sebaceous gland activity, with the resulting sebum production triggering hyperkeratosis. This process blocks the follicle and results in dilation and the ultimate formation of a comedone. The transition from comedone to lesion is due to an inflammatory cascade being triggered, most likely the bacteria *Propionibacterium acnes*.

The most common health condition linked with acne lesions (in women) is polycystic ovarian syndrome (PCOS). Confirmation of a PCOS diagnosis is difficult to ascertain because it involves similar biological markers to acne vulgaris such as elevated testosterone and insulin resistance. However, women with PCOS also present with other symptoms such as hirsutism, weight gain and menstrual irregularities. There is also a possibility that acne lesions may be linked to steroidal hormones such as testosterone or corticosteroids.

MEDICAL CONDITIONS THAT MAY MIMIC OR AGGRAVATE ACNE VULGARIS SYMPTOMS

- Papulopustular rosacea
- Perioral dermatitis
- Gram-negative infection
- Steroid acne
- Polycystic ovarian syndrome
- Bacterial folliculitis
- Hidradenitis suppurativa
- Miliaria
- Pseudofolliculitis barbae
- Seborrhoeic dermatitis

Treatment protocol

- The approach to treatment is to improve metabolite clearance and reduce the effect of exacerbating factors while providing agents to reduce inflammation and promote connective tissue healing.

- The herbal formula as shown in the treatment box includes herbs selected due to their anti-inflammatory (*Centella asiatica* and *Calendula officinalis*), depurative (*Centella asiatica*), adaptogenic (*Centella asiatica* and *Schisandra chinensis*), antidepressant (*Hypericum perforatum* and *Schisandra chinensis*) and nervine tonic activity (*Hypericum perforatum*, *Schisandra chinensis* and *Centella asiatica*).

- Further support of the internal herbal formula is provided through the topical wash consisting of *Calendula officinalis* (for its vulnerary and antibacterial activity), *Calendula sinensis* (as a topical anti-inflammatory) and *Melaleuca alternifolia* (due to its antimicrobial activity).

- The treatment aims are also supported with a nutritional formula containing selenium, vitamin A, vitamin E, bromelains, quercetin and zinc to assist in reducing inflammation and oxidation while promoting connective tissue repair.

- It is vital that this is combined with dietary recommendations to reduce sugar and refined carbohydrate intake and increase consumption of unprocessed grains and whole foods.

- It is also important to encourage a better lifestyle balance, particularly by increasing the amount of time spent on enjoyable activities. This will help reduce the stress response.

PRESCRIPTION
Herbal formula (100 mL)

Calendula officinalis 1:2	20 mL
Centella asiatica 1:2	30 mL
Hypericum perforatum 1:2	25 mL
Schisandra chinensis 1:2	25 mL
Dose: 5 mL 2 × daily	

Nutritional prescription

Quercetin: 400 mg 2 × daily
Bromelains: 100 mg 2 × daily
Zinc (gluconate): 4 mg 2 × daily
Selenium: 13 mcg 2 × daily
Vitamin A: 2500 IU 2 × daily
Vitamin E: 242 IU 2 × daily
1 tablet 2 × daily before meals

Topical wash

1 cup infusion of *Calendula officinalis* (5 g), *Camellia sinensis* (5 g) and *Melaleuca alternifolia* (100% essential oil) (5 drops)
Apply topically using a clean cloth or cotton wool daily

Expected outcomes and follow-up protocols

Symptoms should improve within 1 month, although all lesions may not have cleared. However, concomitant improvements such as reduction in food cravings, improved sleep and better mood can also be expected. With these changes, the herbal formula can be modified to focus more on lymphatic clearance rather than on nervous system support. This can be achieved by replacing *Schisandra chinensis* with an *Echinacea angustifolia/purpurea* blend while maintaining her nutritional supplement and dietary changes.

Within another month, new lesions can be expected to cease, and ongoing treatment can then focus on regulating the hypothalamic–pituitary–adrenal (HPA) axis through adaptogenic herbs such as *Glycyrrhiza glabra*. It is important to develop a prescription plan for acne vulgaris carefully given the younger age of many individuals with the condition. Cooking skills, time commitments and budget all need to be considered. It may take 2–3 months of consistent treatment before results are noticed with acne vulgaris. If blood sugar irregularities become evident through case taking, and basic dietary changes are not addressing them, further investigations may be necessary. Specifically, a glucose tolerance test (with insulin) may identify subacute glucose intolerance or pancreatic insufficiency. If this is the case the treatment regimen will need to be modified to incorporate a stronger focus in this area.

Clinical pearls

- Hormonal imbalance, particularly androgen excess, plays a prominent role in the pathophysiology of acne vulgaris.

- Inflammation is a key consideration in treatment and may be affected by bacterial infection, dietary choices, stress response or hormonal imbalance—treat the underlying factors creating inflammation, as well as using anti-inflammatory treatments.

- It is *always* important to address dietary and lifestyle factors in acne vulgaris management, even if change is made slowly.

Expert | CONSULT

Clinical Comprehension Questions & Answers are hosted on
https://expertconsult.inkling.com/store/book/
sarris-clinical-naturopathy-case-files-1

BIBLIOGRAPHY

Bassett IB, Pannowitz DL, Barnetson RSC. A comparative study of tea-tree oil versus benzoylperoxide in the treatment of acne. *Med J Aust.* 1990;153(8):455-458.

Leach M. The Dermatological System. In: Hechtman L, ed. *Clinical Naturopathic Medicine.* Sydney: Elsevier; 2012.

Smith RN, Mann NJ, Braue A, et al. The effect of a high-protein, low glycemic-load diet versus a conventional, high glycemic-load diet on biochemical parameters associated with acne vulgaris: a randomized, investigator-masked, controlled trial. *J Am Acad Dermatol.* 2007;57:247-256.

Spencer EH, Ferdowsian HR, Barnard ND. Diet and acne: a review of the evidence. *Int J Dermatol.* 2009;48(4):339-347.

Steel A. Inflammatory Skin Disorders—Atopic Eczema and Psoriasis. In: Sarris J, Wardle J, eds. *Clinical Naturopathy: an Evidence-Based Guide to Practice.* Sydney: Elsevier; 2014.

36 Eczema and psoriasis

Amie Steel

PRESENTATION

A 32-year-old female office worker presents to the clinic with **previously diagnosed eczema**. She has **dry, scaly patches** around her **mouth, fingers** and on the **inside of her elbows**. They are very **red, itchy and papular** and are only relieved by using low-perfume moisturisers and steroidal creams. They appear to be **aggravated by stress and the change of seasons**. She was initially diagnosed with eczema at 5 years old; this has persisted for most of her life. This patient **does not report feeling any hunger signal** but finds that she **craves sweets**. Her **flatus is 'offensive'** and worse when she eats meat products. She moves her bowels every 1 or 2 days, but her motions are small and unformed.

Diagnostic considerations

As most eczema and psoriasis is diagnosed based on the appearance of the lesions it is important to verify whether the patient's immunity is dominated by the innate or adaptive immunity. Regardless of the skin condition diagnosis given, it is the immune balance that should drive internal treatments. It is also important to explore the gastrointestinal function in patients presenting with skin disorders to identify whether dysbiosis or other related conditions are contributing to the clinical picture.

Atopic dermatitis (eczema) is most frequently diagnosed in infancy but may continue into the adult years. It involves an inherited tendency towards type 1 hypersensitivity reactions, and, as such, it is common to also see eczema or other allergic conditions (such as allergic rhinitis and asthma) in a person's family history. The physiological response to the allergen causes chronic inflammation and requires pathology testing for conclusive diagnosis.

The pathophysiology of psoriasis is complex and involves immunological pathways and genetic susceptibility. It has been mostly linked with increased cellular proliferation and hyperkeratinisation of the dermal layer, although this feature is believed to be preceded by leucocyte infiltration. It is believed that these T-cells remain activated and cause the skin to constantly regenerate, and for this reason psoriasis is categorised as an autoimmune condition.

Like eczema, psoriasis also begins with small red papules, but lesions eventually develop a silvery plaque (although the basal layer remains red and inflamed). Most commonly, psoriatic lesions are seen on the face, scalp, elbow and knees. Another potentially important intracellular compound is cyclic-AMP (cAMP), which is understood to regulate cellular proliferation, although the precise mechanism and resulting effect on psoriasis are still unclear.

MEDICAL CONDITIONS THAT MAY PRESENT WITH DERMATITIS SYMPTOMS

- Eczema (atopic and contact dermatitis)
- Psoriasis
- Tinea
- Stevens-Johnson syndrome
- Toxic epidermal necrolysis
- Erythema multiforme major
- Drug rash with eosinophilia and systemic symptoms
- Candida intertrigo
- Erythrasma
- Dermatophyte infection
- Annular erythemas
- Lupus erythematosus
- Lichen planus
- Pityriasis rosea and versicolor

Treatment protocol

- If not undertaken previously, the initial prescription for this case involves allergy testing. In this case an immunoglobulin E (IgE) test is advised.
- It is important to not prescribe strong antihistamine or immune-modulating interventions prior to allergy testing because this may skew the results.
- Omega-3 fatty acids (especially high-EPA formulations) and mixed probiotics including strains of *Lactobacillus rhamnosus* and *Lactobacillus plantarum* can be included initially until any dietary or environmental allergens have been identified.
- Vitamin D supplementation may be an appropriate adjuvant therapy with the probiotics. The need for this nutrient may be indicated due to her occupational status (working long hours indoors).

- General dietary recommendations to reduce common allergens such as cow's milk and wheat may also be useful.

PRESCRIPTION

Nutritional prescription

Omega-3 fish oil: 3 × 1000 mg capsules with breakfast

Probiotic complex (containing *Lactobacillus rhamnosus*): ½ tsp [equivalent to 10 × 10^9 organisms]

Vitamin D: 2000 IU daily

Investigations

Specific IgE test

Expected outcomes and follow-up protocols

Upon receipt of the IgE allergy profile results, dietary modifications can be undertaken to reduce her intake of allergenic foods. Beyond this, modifying the initial prescription to focus on addressing possible intestinal hyperpermeability may be indicated. This can include *Saccharomyces boulardii* and a prebiotic formula containing glutamine (an important energy substrate for enterocytes) as well as *Ulmus rubra* and pectin. Further digestive support to stimulate gastric acid and support protein digestion, such as *Gentiana lutea*, may also be useful at this stage, depending on the patient's presenting condition. If preferred, antihistamine herbs (such as *Albizia lebbeck*) may be included in the treatment. Alternatively, it may be worth waiting to see if the antihistamine activity is necessary once the allergens have been removed from the diet.

After 4–8 weeks of intestinal repair, it is beneficial to revisit previous triggers such as stress and provide HPA support (such as *Eleutherococcus senticosus* and *Rhodiola rosea*) to ameliorate the effect this has on the immune system. It is possible to have initiated treatment with immune-modulating herbs such as *Hemidesmus indicus*, *Albizia lebbeck* or *Echinacea angustifolia*, but this is only appropriate if allergy testing is not being performed. Any testing that is being undertaken to determine baseline physiological activity must not be masked by potent therapeutic interventions such as herbal or high-dose nutritional supplementation. Also, given the weight of evidence that suggests the potential benefit of probiotics in managing this condition, it is proposed that using these interventions initially allows for a clear measure of their efficacy in the individual case. It then allows the practitioner to consider other interventions to address additional contributing aspects of the patient's health rather than as a focus of treatment. Remember that, because a person can only take on so many prescribed products at any one time, ensuring that the prescription is most effective in the long run is important.

Clinical pearls

- Ensure that, where possible, any allergenic triggers are removed as a primary step in management.
- Pay close attention to any signs of dysbiosis and treat accordingly.
- Provide lifestyle support to reduce the stress response.
- Avoid using any immune-modulating interventions prior to testing for antigens as this may mask results.

Expert | CONSULT

Clinical Comprehension Questions & Answers are hosted on
**https://expertconsult.inkling.com/store/book/
sarris-clinical-naturopathy-case-files-1**

BIBLIOGRAPHY

Boyle RJ, Bath-Hextall FJ, Leonardi-Bee J, et al. Probiotics for treating eczema (review). *Cochrane Database Syst Rev.* 2008;(1):CD006135.

Harvima IT, Nilsson G. Stress, the neuroendocrine system and mast cells: current understanding of their role in psoriasis. *Expert Rev Clin Immunol.* 2012;8:235-241.

Ly NP, Litonjua A, Gold DR, et al. Gut microbiota, probiotics, and vitamin D: interrelated exposures influencing allergy, asthma, and obesity? *J Allergy Clin Immunol.* 2011;127(5).1087-1094.

Steel A. Inflammatory skin disorders – atopic eczema and psoriasis. In: Sarris J, Wardle J, eds. *Clinical Naturopathy: An Evidence-Based Guide to Practice.* 2nd ed. Sydney: Churchill Livingstone; 2014.

Viljanen M, Pohjavuori E, Haahtela T, et al. Induction of inflammation as a possible mechanism of probiotic effect in atopic eczema-dermatitis syndrome. *J Allergy Clin Immunol.* 2005;115:1254-1259.

Wright RJ, Cohen RT, Cohen S. The impact of stress on the development and expression of atopy. *Curr Opin Allergy Clin Immunol.* 2005;5:23-29.

37 | Hormonal acne

Kathleen Murphy

PRESENTATION

A 29-year-old female presents with **premenstrual syndrome (PMS)** and **mild hormonal acne** following cessation of the oral contraceptive pill (OCP) 8 weeks ago. **For the past 6 years, she has taken a low-dose combined OCP**. She has a **history of cystic acne** on her chin and neck, which was severe in her late teens and early 20s, but controlled with OCP use.

The patient is newly married and has gone off the pill to prepare for conception. She works in the beauty industry and is concerned about her 'problem skin' returning and its impact professionally. Since ceasing the OCP, the patient has had one cycle, with a light period that lasted 3 days. **In the week prior and during her menstrual period, the patient felt extremely emotional (tearful, anxious and irritable) and developed inflamed comedones and papules on her chin**. Although she feels that her emotions return to normal after her period, the patient's skin has remained inflamed around her chin and jawline. She is currently at day 15 of her cycle.

The patient is also training for a marathon and runs a minimum of 10 km most mornings. Her stress about her work, hormones and appearance have made her more sensitive and resulted in tension with her husband over the past month. She has a body mass index of 20 and **often craves sweet foods**, particularly when stressed. Tests reveal that her **vitamin D levels are suboptimal**. Results of a sex hormone profile are pending. All other parameters appear normal.

Diagnostic considerations

Management of this case should focus on re-establishing a natural cycle by regulating her reproductive hormones, taking into account factors such as the patient's stress levels, lifestyle practices and diagnosed deficiencies. PMS and other symptoms that synchronise with the menstrual cycle, including acne, involve complex interactions between ovarian hormones, endogenous opioids, neurotransmitters, prostaglandins and endocrine systems. As such, successful management will require more than hormonal adjustment alone.

As the patient has only recently transitioned off oral contraception after years of continuous use, it is pertinent to consider the liver's role in the emotional and physical symptoms she presents with. It is also important to include vitamin D in this picture, as it plays an important role in both hormone regulation and the inflammation cascade.

The patient exercises heavily, and frequent high-intensity exercise places significant physiological stress on the body. This promotes inflammation and compromises adrenal function, in turn affecting regulation of the hypothalamic–pituitary–ovarian (HPO) axis and affecting the reproductive cycle.

The patient's nutritional status must also be considered in managing this case and a thorough assessment conducted. Certain dietary factors are implicated in the presence of hormone-related acne, including excessive milk consumption and foods with a high glycaemic load (e.g. refined, sweetened and highly processed foods). It's important to eliminate those foods known to aggravate symptoms while increasing the intake of foods that reduce inflammation and promote normal healthy skin function.

The patient's symptoms are also suggestive of polycystic ovarian syndrome and referral for further investigation may be warranted to ensure correct diagnosis.

OTHER CONDITIONS TO ASSESS FOR

- Polycystic ovarian syndrome
- Affective disorder such as anxiety or depression
- Personality disorder
- Acne vulgaris
- Rosacea
- Perioral dermatitis

Treatment protocol

- Re-establishing a healthy cycle is the goal of treatment, and an important aspect of this is teaching the patient to reconnect with her body's natural rhythm after years of medication. Menstrual charting—for at least three full cycles—is an excellent tool for this purpose and will help the patient monitor the length of her cycle, the symptoms that occur throughout and other factors that may be influencing this.

- *Vitex agnus-castus* may be considered to relieve symptoms of PMS and promote healthy ovulation.

- Optimal liver metabolism should be encouraged with hepatic herbs such as *Silybum marianum* and *Bupleurum falcatum*. The nutritional compound diindolylmethane (DIM) could also be considered to encourage better hormone clearance.

- Alterative or depurative herbs can help to cleanse the system and relieve inflammatory skin symptoms. Examples include *Urtica dioica* and *Arctium lappa*.
- Zinc supplementation would be appropriate to reduce the severity of skin inflammation and promote healing, and to support hormone metabolism and neurotransmitter function.
- Modulating the stress response is an important consideration for this patient and can include the use of adaptogenic herbs such as *Withania somnifera* and *Schisandra chinensis*, as well as nutrients that support nervous system function such as magnesium and B vitamins. It would also be beneficial to replace several high-intensity exercise sessions each week with more restful, low-impact activity alongside mindfulness practice.
- Dietary advice should include recommendations for adequate protein, whole grains, fresh fruit and vegetables and good fats in order to stabilise blood sugar and maximise nutrient intake. Consumption of sugar, caffeine and alcohol should be limited or avoided as these may promote inflammation and exacerbate emotional symptoms of PMS.
- Essential fatty acids should also be increased through the diet and supplementation considered. These play an important role in hormone synthesis, inflammation and mental/emotional health.

PRESCRIPTION

Herbal formula (100 mL)

Withania somnifera 1:2	25 mL
Schisandra chinensis 1:2	25 mL
Silybum marianum 1:1	25 mL
Bupleurum falcatum 1:2	25 mL

7.5 mL morning and evening

Vitex agnus-castus tablet (standardised): 1 tablet daily, on rising

Nutritional prescription

Vitamin D: 1000 IU—2 capsules daily with food

Omega-3 fish oil: 1000 mg—2 capsules daily with food

Multivitamin B complex—1 tablet with breakfast

Zinc: 20 mg elemental—1 tablet 2 × daily with food

Lifestyle prescription

Dietary improvement

Urtica dioica leaf tea: 2 cups daily

Reduce high-intensity exercise in favour of low-impact activity

Appropriate sun exposure to encourage vitamin D synthesis

Expected outcomes and follow-up protocol

An initial review would be recommended within 2 weeks of the first consultation to ensure patient compliance and to follow up on any change in symptoms over that time. However, due to the fact that the patient's complaints are tied to her menstrual cycle, it is important to allow at least three full cycles to monitor the patient's progress before considering significant change to her treatment regimen.

Although the patient may experience noticeable improvement within her first cycle, it is also possible that the condition will change very little, or worsen, before exhibiting noticeable symptom reduction. For this reason, monthly follow-ups are recommended in the first 3–6 months following the start of treatment. During this time, necessary adjustments can be made to the prescription as required and recommendations for dietary and lifestyle changes given as appropriate. Where there continues to be no significant improvement, or symptoms continually worsen, referral for additional pathology and biochemical testing is warranted.

Clinical pearls

- Menstrual complaints are not only related to reproductive hormones but can be influenced by a number of body systems.

- Menstrual complaints aren't the only symptoms of hormonal dysfunction.

- All types of stress—mental/emotional and physical—have a significant impact on hormonal regulation and inflammatory conditions and therefore need to be addressed in treatment.

Expert | CONSULT

Clinical Comprehension Questions & Answers are hosted on **https://expertconsult.inkling.com/store/book/ sarris-clinical-naturopathy-case-files-1**

BIBLIOGRAPHY

Albuquerque R, Rocha MA, Bagatin E, et al. Could adult female acne be associated with modern life? *Arch Dermatol Res.* 2014;306(8):683-688.

Bianco V, Cestari AM, Casati D, et al. Premenstrual syndrome and beyond: lifestyle, nutrition, and personal facts. *Minerva Ginecol.* 2014;66(4):365-375.

Leach M. The dermatological system. In: Hechtman L, ed. *Clinical Naturopathic Medicine.* Sydney: Elsevier; 2012.

Steel A. Acne vulgaris. In: Sarris J, Wardle J, eds. *Clinical Naturopathy: An Evidence-Based Guide to Practice.* 2nd ed. Sydney: Elsevier; 2014.

Trickey R. *Women, Hormones and the Menstrual Cycle.* Fairfield: Trickey Enterprises; 2011.

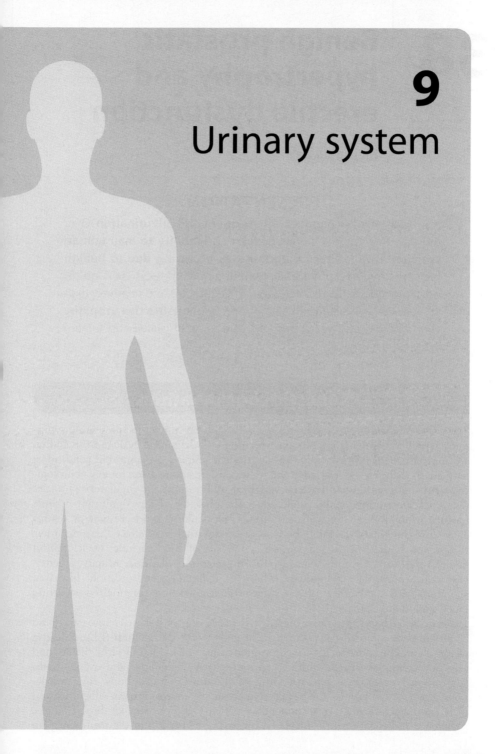

9

Urinary system

Benign prostatic hypertrophy and erectile dysfunction

Kieran Cooley

PRESENTATION

A 55-year-old male presents with **frequent difficult urination**. Over the past few months he has noticed an **inability to maintain an erection**. This has been **diagnosed as occurring due to benign prostatic hypertrophy (BPH)**. His body mass index is 26.5 and his waist:hip ratio is 1.2. His diet is low in vegetables and relatively high in red meat. In his early 40s he suffered from **obstructive uropathy** over a period of 2 years; this was due to renal calculi and treated using ultrasound.

Diagnostic considerations

The initial case-taking process should assess the clinical state of the presenting symptoms as well as involving a thorough screening and diagnostic evaluation including a complete patient history. This is to identify the presence of comorbid conditions, particularly diabetes, dyslipidaemia and hypertension, and to assess for any neurological, structural (i.e. lumbar or sacral vertebral subluxations) or circulatory obstacles to proper innervation of the pelvic area. The presence of any significant organic (circulatory or a side effects of medications, particularly antidepressant or neurogenic), psychosomatic or mind–body connections that may affect these disorders should also be investigated. Suggestive symptoms of BPH include: weak, painful or incomplete micturition; acute or chronic retention of urine; urinary urgency, particularly nocturnal; inability to achieve or maintain a full erection; increased abdominal mass and other cardiovascular risk factors; and potential co-occurring mood and libido changes.

An evidence-based integrative prescriptive plan using a risk-based approach should be provided to comprehensively treat BPH and erectile dysfunction (ED). Lifestyle factors should be addressed and incorporated as part of normal, healthy dietary and exercise patterns consistent with the patient's state, capabilities and overall goals. Motivational issues, their understanding of the disease and options, time restrictions, financial limitations, the perspective about the source of their difficulties and their treatment priorities, may influence a patient's ability to make those changes. Adherence and engagement is increased by having ownership of the treatment plan and a sense of shared partnership in its development and planning. Due to this, all treatment strategies should be developed considering the above factors, and the management and treatment strategy should be individually tailored and offered in a step-wise manner, incorporating appropriate follow-up and monitoring of the disease state. General lifestyle advice should focus on encouraging a balance between meaningful work, adequate rest and sleep, judicious exercise, positive social and sexual interactions and pleasurable hobbies. If substance abuse or other significant biopsychosocial challenges exist, these need to be discussed and incorporated as part of treatment or referral to other effective healthcare providers or existing services.

MEDICAL CONDITIONS THAT MAY MIMIC OR AGGRAVATE BPH

- Carcinoma of the bladder
- Cystitis (infection or radiation induced)
- Foreign bodies in the bladder (stones or retained stents) or bladder trauma
- Pelvic floor dysfunction or chronic pelvis pain (prostatodynia)
- Prostatitis or prostatic abscess
- Prostate cancer
- Overactive bladder or neurogenic bladder
- Spinal or pelvic structural abnormalities, vertebral subluxations or conditions that affect nerve innervation to the pelvic region
- Urethral stricture due to trauma or a sexually transmitted disease
- Urinary tract infection

Treatment protocol

- The patient should be advised to increase physical activity, including a mix of aerobic and anaerobic activity for at least 30 minutes three times per week to address mood, weight loss, blood flow and cardiovascular risk.

- The treatment rationale of herbal and nutritional supplementation is aimed at regulating androgens and addressing inflammation using a relatively high dose of *Serenoa repens*, Cernilton, *Pygeum africanum* and zinc.

- Urinary tract symptoms are addressed using *Urtica dioica*.

- A tablespoon of flaxseed oil twice a day will address inflammation and cardiovascular risk markers.

- Dietary advice includes consuming a diet high in soluble fibre to help address cardiovascular risk and regulate weight, 100 g of soy products (soybeans or tofu) each day to assist hormone regulation, and to increase fruit consumption to facilitate hydroxylation and elimination of dihydro-testosterone (DHT).

- The patient should be advised that the urogenital health of his partner is necessary for a healthy sexual relationship.
- Other prescriptive options include increased consumption of pumpkin seeds, which are sources of essential fatty acids and zinc. Limit alcohol consumption, particularly beer.
- Acute catheterisation may be necessary if urine outflow is sufficiently obstructed, or co-management using alpha-blockers to address symptoms that significantly affect quality of life (nocturia and urinary frequency).

PRESCRIPTION
Herbal formula (100 mL)

Urtica dioica (radix) 1:2	35 mL
Epilobium spp. 1:2	35 mL
Pygeum africanum 1:2	30 mL

Dose: 5 mL 3 × daily
Serenoa repens tablets: 160 mg 2 × daily
Flower pollen extract (e.g. Cernilton) 63 mg 2–3 × daily

Nutritional prescription

Flaxseed oil: 1 tbsp 2 × daily
Zinc amino acid chelate: 50 mg/day
High-fibre diet including 100 g of soy products each day

Expected outcomes and follow-up protocols

Regulation of androgens and hormones may take up to 2 months, and patients may need additional or integrative support to manage symptoms while addressing the root cause. If prostate-specific antigen (PSA) levels are used as one means of monitoring prostate health, this test should be done once every 6 months (especially if there is a significantly enlarged prostate on digital rectal exam). BPH symptoms should be reassessed every 6 weeks if moderate, and at least every 4 weeks if severe. Patients can keep a diary of daily trips to the toilet, fluid intake and attempts to collect urine output, as a means of assessing the effectiveness of treatment as well as whether adjunctive or emergency care is warranted.

Improvements to ED may take time, particularly if there is a strong psychological component, and a discussion with the patient that encourages realistic expectations for changes but that adds no undue pressure should take place. Individual or couples counselling may be warranted. If the root cause of BPH and ED is likely to be vascular in origin, and there are no signs or diagnostic tests indicating hypertension, infection, hormone abnormalities or inflammation, 3 g/day of L-arginine could improve ED as well as circulation. If no improvements occur within 3 months, other therapeutic options include removing the potential sources of inflammation in the diet, supplementation using glycine, alanine and glutamic acid (6 g/day), and the use of herbal medicines such as *Epilobium* spp. for BPH and *Ginkgo biloba* or *Tribulus terrestris* for ED.

Clinical pearls

- BPH shares many properties with cardiovascular, metabolic syndrome, ED, depression and urinary tract infection disorders.

- The holistic treatment approach should look beyond hormonal regulation and include therapies to reduce inflammation, reduce oxidative stress and improve nitric oxide production.

- BPH is predominantly an androgen-mediated disorder. Factors that decrease the production of DHT should be included in most treatment protocols.

- Counselling to address issues of ageing, mood and sexual health may be important in moderating quality of life and the mental/emotional aspects of these diseases.

Expert | CONSULT

Clinical Comprehension Questions & Answers are hosted on
https://expertconsult.inkling.com/store/book/
sarris-clinical-naturopathy-case-files-1

BIBLIOGRAPHY

Cooley K. Benign prostatic hypertrophy. In: Sarris J, Wardle J, eds. *Clinical Naturopathy: An Evidence-Based Guide to Practice*. 2nd ed. Sydney: Elsevier; 2014.

Moyad MA, Barada JH, Lue TF, et al. Prevention and treatment of erectile dysfunction using lifestyle changes and dietary supplements: what works and what is worthless, parts 1 and 2. *Uro Clin N Am*. 2004;31:249-273.

Roehrborn CG. Benign prostatic hyperplasia and lower urinary tract symptom guidelines. *Can Urol Assoc J*. 2012;6(5 suppl 2):S130-S132.

Rosenberg MT. Diagnosis and management of erectile dysfunction in the primary care setting. *Int J Clin Prac*. 2007;61(7):1198-1208.

Zakaria L, Anastasiadis AG, Shabsigh R. Common conditions of the aging male: erectile dysfunction, benign prostatic hyperplasia, cardiovascular disease and depression. *Int Urol Nephrol*. 2001;33(2):283-292.

Zhu YS, Imperato-McGinley JL. 5 alpha-reductase isozymes and androgen actions in the prostate. *Ann N Y Acad Sci*. 2009;1155:43-56.

39 Recurrent urinary tract infections

Michelle Boyd

PRESENTATION

A 33-year-old female presents with **chronic, recurrent urinary tract infections** (UTIs) (specifically cystitis) that have affected her all her adult life. They have been previously treated but not resolved with antibiotic treatment. She currently reports **extreme pain and discomfort upon urination**. No blood appears in her urine. She mentions that it seems to get **worse after she has sex**. She is also susceptible to 'whatever is going around' and usually suffers from **at least two or three colds/flu each year**, especially around the change of seasons and winter months. She works full time as an office manager and complains of **mental fatigue**, especially in the afternoon.

Diagnostic considerations

Treatment will focus on symptomatic relief (urination pain) and reducing the incidence, frequency and long-term complications (scarring and kidney disease) of recurrent UTIs, as well as reducing the incidence of colds/flu. It may incorporate herbal medicine, probiotics and diet and lifestyle advice. To identify the most appropriate treatment options, focus should be given to promoting the body's natural UTI defence mechanisms including: improving flow and volume of urine—stagnation can increase adherence of bacteria, and infective bacteria can be 'flushed out' by increasing urine volume (using diuretic teas and increasing water intake); promoting painless urination (using urinary demulcents and anti-inflammatories); facilitating complete bladder emptying and improving bladder tone (using a spasmolytic to reduce lower bladder sphincter resistance and a 'bladder tonic'); reducing bacterial adherence to the bladder wall; and enhancing the patient's immune defences to appropriately remove and resist infection. In some situations—notably pregnancy—UTIs can escalate quite quickly, with serious consequences. These should be monitored with additional caution.

Various dietary and lifestyle factors also need to be explored to deduce the patient's susceptibility to and incidence of UTIs and to promote general wellbeing and healthy immune function. The consultation should target identifying and reducing or eliminating exacerbating influences that may irritate the bladder epithelial tissue, predisposing the patient to infection and hindering treatment effects (these may include caffeine, refined sugars, dietary allergens, alcohol and nicotine). Non-organic retail meats like chicken and pork should also be discouraged due to antimicrobial-resistant UTI-causing *E. coli* found in these foods and being transferred via faeces to the urogenital area.

The importance of hydration for mental and physical health should be considered; water requirements can be underestimated and even the mildest dehydration can imbalance the homeostatic function of our internal environment. The temperature of our environment (whether outdoors in the summer heat or indoors in air-conditioning), our physical activity and alcohol consumption all promote dehydration. Water requirements fluctuate with air temperature and our metabolic rate (activity level). Most fluids should be consumed away from meals so digestive juices are not diluted. Further considerations need to be made for previous antibiotic use and any resistance patterns that may have resulted from this, along with possible development of microbial imbalance/dysbiosis and the long-term effect this may have on gut health and related inflammation/immune system dysfunction.

MEDICAL CONDITIONS THAT MAY MIMIC OR AGGRAVATE RECURRENT UTIS

- Acute pyelonephritis*
- Interstitial cystitis
- Genital herpes
- Atrophic vaginitis
- Bladder cancer

*Suspected pyelonephritis requires urgent medical attention. Apart from common UTI symptoms (e.g. painful, burning, urgent and/or frequent urination), pyelonephritis presents with more severe symptoms including back pain, fever or chills, and nausea and vomiting.

Treatment protocol

- *Vaccinium macrocarpon* provides an antibacterial and antiadhesive effect, preventing bacteria (*E. coli*) from adhering to the uroepithelial cell wall and further preventing proliferation throughout the urinary tract.
- *Echinacea angustifolia* is prescribed to enhance immune-modulating activity.
- The herbal medicinal tea prescribed (detailed in the prescription box) enhances hydration, increases urine volume and diuresis, provides soothing demulcent effects and enhances the anti-inflammatory and antiseptic actions. *Mentha x piperita* is a spasmolytic and antimicrobial and enhances flavour (taste of tea), and with *Agathosma betulina* provides a pleasant aromatic experience. *Solidago virgaurea* is an anti-inflammatory and promotes

diuresis (without promoting loss of electrolytes). *Althaea officinalis* provides a soothing demulcent.

- Probiotics are prescribed to rebalance the microflora (possibly due to previous antibiotic use) and enhance immune defences. Specifically proven *Lactobacillus* strains include *L. rhamnosus* GR-1 and *L. reuteri* RC-14.

- Dietary and lifestyle advice includes advising the patient to eat regularly and especially include afternoon tea to ensure adequate blood sugar levels are maintained throughout the working afternoon. Fructo-oligosaccharide-containing foods like onions, garlic, Jerusalem artichokes and banana can be included, as should probiotic foods such as cultured yoghurts. She should avoid refined sugars, stimulants and non-organic meats.

PRESCRIPTION
Herbal prescription

Vaccinium macrocarpon capsules (equivalent to 300 mL *Vaccinium macrocarpon* juice, standardised for 36 mg proanthocyanidins): 1 capsule each morning
Echinacea angustifolia 1 g tablets (standardised for alkylamides): 1 tablet 3 × daily

Herbal tea

100 g dried herb mix containing:
Agathosma betulina leaf 20 g
Zea mays styles and stigmas 20 g
Solidago virgaurea aerial parts 10 g
Arctostaphylos uva-ursi leaf 15 g
Althaea officinalis root 15 g
Mentha x piperita leaf 20 g

Preparation

15 g infused in covered vessel (teapot) for 15 minutes
1 cup 3 × daily on an empty stomach on rising, mid-afternoon and before bed (prepare each morning for use throughout the day)
Probiotics capsules containing minimum of 20 billion organisms in a blend including *Lactobacillus rhamnosus* GR-1, *L. reuteri* RC-14, *L. casei shirota* and *L. crispatus* CTV-05: 2 capsules daily with dinner

Lifestyle prescription

Ensure adequate hydration and urination
Remove dietary irritants
Incorporate pre- and probiotic foods in the diet
Practise urogenital hygiene

- Advise the patient about the importance of maintaining hydration for treating and preventing UTIs—a minimum of 3 L clean water daily, preferably consumed away from meals.

- The patient should also be advised about the importance of urogenital hygiene and urination (by both sexual partners) before and after sexual activity, and to always cleanse the urogenital and anal areas from front to back.

Expected outcomes and follow-up protocols

Relief would be expected within a few days of starting the prescription. Increased immune resistance and improved balance in the bowel and of urogenital flora will reduce UTI occurrence. Furthermore, a reduced occurrence rate should follow, particularly if the diet and lifestyle advice is followed.

A follow-up appointment should be scheduled for 4 weeks after starting the prescription. If all goes to plan, supply a further 3 months' prescription for continued preventative measures: adhering to previous diet and lifestyle advice; a prophylactic prescription of *Echinacea angustifolia* (to improve immune defences); and *Vaccinium macrocarpon* to promote continued urinary tract health by preventing adherence/proliferation of any opportunistic pathogenic *E. coli* to uroepithelial cells.

Clinical pearls

- UTIs are common, especially in young women, and the recurrence rate is high.

- UTIs are associated with increased risk of other urinary tract conditions such as pyelonephritis (a red flag), so should be treated assertively and comprehensively.

- Antibiotic treatment of UTIs may lead to patterns of antibiotic resistance, so judicious use is advised and use of clinically proven alternative treatments should be considered.

- Various herbal and nutritional therapeutics have value in treating and preventing UTIs and can be considered as stand-alone interventions or adjuvants with antibiotics.

- Gastrointestinal health and microbial balance must be considered in patients with urinary tract complaints.

- Implementation of lifestyle advice (e.g. urogenital hygiene) is advised to help prevent recurrence.

- A note to practitioners for preparing the herbal tea blend: Herbs can be combined and mixed in a blender to reduce particle size. This improves the extraction of the therapeutic compounds from the infusion process.

Expert | CONSULT

Clinical Comprehension Questions & Answers are hosted on
https://expertconsult.inkling.com/store/book/
sarris-clinical-naturopathy-case-files-1

BIBLIOGRAPHY

Boyd M. Recurrent urinary tract infections. In: Sarris J, Wardle J, eds. *Clinical Naturopathy: An Evidence-Based Guide to Practice*. ed 2. Sydney: Elsevier; 2014.

Falagas ME, Betsi GI, Tokas T, et al. Probiotics for prevention of recurrent urinary tract infections in women. *Drugs*. 2006;66(9):1253-1261.

Gerber SG, Brendler CB. *Evaluation of the Urologic Patient: History, Physical Examination, and Urinalysis. Campbell-Walsh Urology*. 10th ed. Philadelphia: Elsevier Saunders; 2012.

Howell AB, Botto H, Combescure C, et al. Dosage effect on uropathogenic *Escherichia coli* anti-adhesion activity in urine following consumption of cranberry powder standardized for proanthocyanidin content: a multicentric randomized double blind study. *BMC Infect Dis*. 2010;10(94).

Popkin BM, D'Anci KE, Rosenberg IR. Water, hydration and health. *Nutr Rev*. 2010;68(8):439-458.

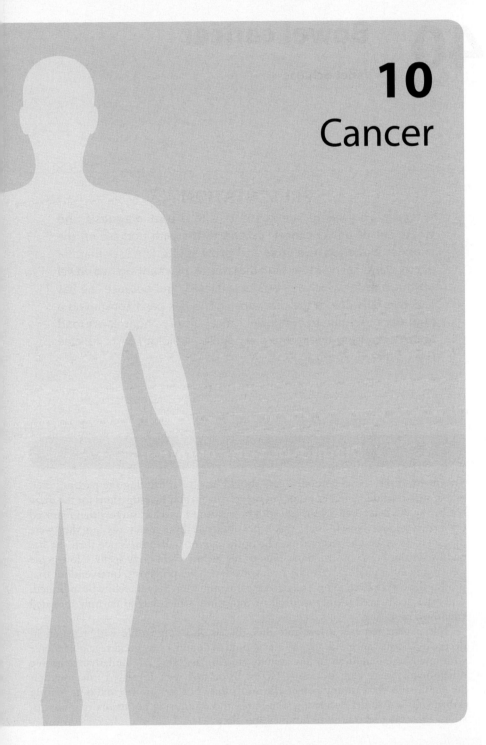

10
Cancer

40 Bowel cancer

Janet Schloss

PRESENTATION

A female, 76 years of age, presents with a **past diagnosis and treatment of bowel cancer**, **osteoarthritis** with nodules on the knuckles, **bowel obstructions** and **dizzy spells**. She says that her doctor wants her on a **low-fibre diet** due to experiencing two bowel obstructions for which she was hospitalised, and because she has had **two falls** due to the dizzy spells. She has been consuming a **high-fibre diet** due to her bowel cancer history and is **concerned about exercising** due to the dizzy spells. Pathology tests indicate she is otherwise healthy.

Diagnostic considerations

Treatment of the abovementioned case should involve addressing the patient's diet, taking into consideration her history of bowel cancer, and investigations for the dizzy spells. She was diagnosed 3 years ago with bowel cancer and had surgery that removed 60% of her lower bowel. There was a possibility of liver metastasis but they were diagnosed as cysts. She received no chemotherapy or radiation. Since then she has had two major bowel obstructions. Due to her arthritis and dizzy spells, a low-grade underlying inflammatory state may be involved with her prognosis. Interventions that protect the bowel, liver, joints and decrease inflammation may therefore be indicated. The dizzy spells need further medical investigation, which has so far only included vitamin B12 testing.

This patient requires a low-fibre diet that is also compatible with research in decreasing bowel cancer. Ideally the diet should maintain a very good vegetable intake with low fibre in addition to low animal protein. Assessing any underlying chronic inflammatory state and decreasing factors associated with increased inflammation are required to decrease any potential stimulation of cancer growth and potentiating arthritis. This includes decreasing stimulants and optimising her mental response to stress, increasing relaxation techniques and sleep.

IMPORTANT DIAGNOSTIC/CLINICAL CONSIDERATIONS

- Diverticulitis
- Small bowel obstruction
- Pancreatitis
- Pelvic inflammatory disease
- Inflammation
- Gallstones
- Benign paroxysmal positional vertigo
- Ménière's disease
- Migraine/headache
- Brain tumour/secondaries
- Vestibular neuronitis

Treatment protocol

- The primary approach is to provide an optimal diet and lifestyle to decrease the risk of the bowel cancer returning or metastasising. In addition, the risk of bowel obstruction also needs to be taken into consideration. This involves a low-fibre diet, which is contradictory to research based on preventing bowel cancer. This includes including low-fibre vegetables such as potatoes, sweet potato, pumpkin, zucchini and squash, which all need to be peeled and well cooked. Fruits include pawpaw, melons, well-cooked fruits with no skin or pips, and for grains it is white rice and products made from white rice. To assist the vegetable intake, prepare a vegetable juice using a powered juicer that removes the fibre and involves cabbage in the mix. In addition, include fish (omega-3 fatty acids), chicken and eggs for protein. Avoiding alcohol is recommended. Maintaining calcium intake is also important because calcium (in addition to vitamin D3) has been shown to be inversely correlated with risks of bowel cancer.

- *Curcuma longa* has been found to aid in the epigenic regulation of human colorectal adenocarcinoma HT-29 cells. Therefore it has the potential to inhibit cell growth in addition to decreasing inflammation.

- Exercise needs to be under supervision due to the dizzy episodes. Recommending a gym or engaging an exercise physiologist or personal trainer may be warranted.

- Nutritional supplement considerations include coenzyme Q10 and vitamin D3, probiotics and aged garlic extract. All of these nutrients have been found to assist in colorectal health, with possible protective effects against bowel cancer. Moreover, aged garlic and coenzyme Q10 can assist heart and cardiovascular health, which may be involved with her dizzy spells. Vitamin D3 also requires a blood test to be taken before treatment begins and every 6 months to monitor levels.

- Isoleucine potentially decreases the incidence of liver metastasis from bowel cancer. This was shown in a mice study and in vitro via down regulations of angiogenesis and inhibition of vascular endothelial growth factor (VEGF). No clinical trials have been undertaken to confirm this finding; however, it is considered safe for humans because it does not affect cell viability and could pose to be a novel prophylactic nutrient for preventing liver metastases from bowel cancer.

- Herbal supplementation, which has less scientific evidence for bowel cancer, could involve *Astragalus membranaceus*, *Zingiber officinale*, *Silybum marianum* and *Uncaria tomentosa*. *Astragalus membranaceus* is for strengthening the immune system and for its anti-cancer activity, *Zingiber officinale* is for anti-inflammatory activity, *Silybum marianum* is for assisting liver function and *Uncaria tomentosa* is for anti-inflammatory and anti-cancer activity.

- General lifestyle advice should focus on encouraging a balance between meaningful work, adequate rest and sleep, and pleasurable social interaction and hobbies.

PRESCRIPTION

Herbal formula (100 mL)

Uncaria tomentosa	35 mL
Astragalus membranaceus	30 mL
Silybum marianum	30 mL
Zingiber officinale	5 mL

Dose: 8 mL 2 × daily after food at morning and night

Nutritional prescription

Co-Q10: 150 mg 2–3 times a day with food
Vitamin D3: 2000 IU/day with food
Isoleucine: 200 mg/day on an empty stomach before bed

Lifestyle prescription

Moderate exercise
Good sleep hygiene and mindfulness meditation
Dietary improvement

Expected outcomes and follow-up protocols

In the abovementioned case, a number of issues and unknown conditions may contribute to confounding factors affecting the health of this patient. This patient has always followed a high-vegetable and high-fibre diet due to her bowel cancer diagnosis. Because of this, changing to a low-fibre diet may feel contradictory to what is required to prevent secondaries and will be mentally challenging. Further investigations are required to confirm the cause of the dizzy spells, which may have an impact on her outcome and future health and wellbeing. Continual monitoring and modulating the diet and prescription will be required as time and further revelations unfold.

Clinical pearls

- Always assess after a diagnosis of cancer.

- Always treat the individual first rather than the disease.

- Stage the treatment rather than overwhelming the person with everything at once.

- It is estimated that an incidence rate of 15–29% of patients who have undergone a bowel resection from bowel cancer may experience a bowel obstruction. All patients who have had a bowel obstruction are recommended to follow a low-fibre diet. The challenge comes with developing a low-fibre diet that is high in vegetables, low in animal products and that is sustainable and palatable for the patient. Contemplate creative ways of using vegetables by removing the fibre and then creating different dishes.

- Always ensure calcium intake through diet for colorectal patients.

Expert | CONSULT

Clinical Comprehension Questions & Answers are hosted on
**https://expertconsult.inkling.com/store/book/
sarris-clinical-naturopathy-case-files-1**

BIBLIOGRAPHY

Gao Z, Guo B, Gao R, et al. Microbiota disbiosis is associated with colorectal cancer. *Front Microbiol.* 2015;6:20. doi:10.3389/fmicb.2015.00020.

Mehta M, Shike M. Diet and physical activity in the prevention of colorectal cancer. *J Natl Compr Canc Netw.* 2014;12(12):1721-1726.

Murata K, Moriyama M. Isoleucine, an essential amino acid, prevents liver metastases of colon cancer by anti-angiogenesis. *Cancer Res.* 2007;67(7):3263-3268.

Ou J, Carbonero F, Zoetendal EG, et al. Diet, microbiota, and microbial metabolites in colon cancer risk in rural Africans and African Americans. *Am J Clin Nutr.* 2013;98(1):111-120.

Schloss J. Cancer. In: Sarris J, Wardle J, eds. *Clinical Naturopathy: An Evidence-based Guide to Practice.* 2nd ed. Sydney: Elsevier; 2014.

Wactawski-Wende J, Kotchen JM, Anderson GL, et al. Calcium plus vitamin D supplementation and the risk of colorectal cancer. *N Engl J Med.* 2006;354:684-696.

41 Prostate cancer

Janet Schloss

PRESENTATION

A male, 52 years of age, presents with a diagnosis of **prostate cancer**. He has a **prostate-specific antigen (PSA) of 7** with a **Gleason score of 7 (3 + 4)**. At present, he has decided to try 3–6 months of natural therapies before deciding on any medical intervention such as surgery. His **diet consists of meat every day**, mostly red with some chicken, pork and seafood. He **consumes limited vegetables and fruit**, has a mixture of white and wholemeal breads and grains, consumes a lot of dairy and has a lot of business lunches and dinners, which consist of fried foods. He drinks approximately 1 L of water and three or four brewed coffees a day (with one sugar and milk). He has **a few beers on most days** and **smokes approximately 20 cigarettes a day**. His energy is low, experiencing **fatigue** most days. He also has **Hashimoto's disease, high cholesterol** and **high blood pressure**.

Diagnostic considerations

Treatment of this case should involve addressing the patient's diet, lifestyle, physical activity and mental state. This patient has also undergone imaging, with the doctors identifying two contained spots in the prostate. His Gleason score is considered to be prognostic for grade group II (best is ≤ 6, worst is 9–10: a Gleason score of 7, but 4 + 3 is considered to be more aggressive). Another PSA blood pathology test and MRI will be conducted to ascertain his prostate status after he tries the natural approach before any intervention is chosen. Hence there is a window of 3–6 months to obtain optimal health and reduced cancer activity for this patient.

Diet and increasing exercise in addition to his response to stress needs to be addressed. Assessing any underlying chronic inflammatory state and decreasing factors associated with increased inflammation are required to decrease any potential stimulation of cancer growth. This includes decreasing stimulants, optimising his mental response to stress and increasing relaxation techniques and sleep. Assessing his mental response and psychological state regarding his cancer is an important treatment and prognostic factor.

In addition, modulating his hormone response via testosterone and oestrogen are important to potentially decrease further tumour stimulation. Using interventions that modulate the 5-alpha reductase pathway and reduce oestrogen may therefore be indicated. Identifying any heavy metal exposure may also be required for certain patients, particularly those who have exposure through their occupation or past events (e.g. painters, farmers, miners).

His fatigue may also be a reflection of cancer growth, lifestyle and thyroid management. Medical referral for management or pathology tests for thyroid function is recommended in addition to cardiovascular disease status.

KEY ASPECTS TO TARGET TO ASSIST PROSTATE AND GENERAL HEALTH

- Diet
- Physical activity
- Alcohol consumption
- Smoking
- Vitamin D3
- Inflammation
- Immune system
- Stress

Treatment protocol

- The primary approach is to provide an optimal diet and lifestyle to decrease prostate cancer growth. This involves decreasing meat (animal products), dairy, eggs and chicken skin while reducing or eliminating alcohol consumption. He should increase his vegetable intake, eat two or three serves of fruit a day, have cooked tomato with fat and eat an overall fresh whole food diet with decreased processed foods.

- Weight management is important not only for reducing the risk factor but increased weight has also been linked with recurrence or metastasis. Green tea is a potent cancer inhibitor and coffee should be limited to two cups a day. A recent human clinical trial also demonstrated that drinking 8 ounces of pomegranate juice daily stabilised rising PSA levels up to four times longer than normal.

- Cessation of smoking is suggested, and he may need assistance with withdrawal.

- Exercise is a key to treatment, with increased daily activity encouraged in addition to set exercise regimens at least three times a week. This may vary according to the individual and their choice of exercise; however, jumping and quick anaerobic activity has been shown to be effective for preserving bone density.

- Nutritional supplementation considerations include coenzyme Q10 and melatonin—both have been found to lower human prostate cancer cell growth. Vitamin D3 has inhibited prostate cancer growth in several studies. Note: those men without a gall bladder will not absorb supplemental vitamin D3 because it is a fat-soluble vitamin. Nano-particle-based supplements or injections may be required for those patients. In addition, blood tests are required for vitamin D3 before and during supplementation.
- Herbal supplementation has less scientific evidence for prostate cancer but has still been shown to have possible benefits.
- *Pygeum africanum*, curcumin and *Zingiber officinale* can be prescribed. *Pygeum africanum* has anti-cancer properties for prostate cancer in vitro and in vivo, curcumin is for anti-inflammatory and anti-angiogenesis activity and *Zingiber officinale* is for anti-inflammatory activity. Essiac tea has also been used extensively for most cancers.
- General lifestyle advice should focus on encouraging a balance between meaningful work, adequate rest and sleep, and pleasurable social interaction and hobbies.

PRESCRIPTION

Herbal formula

Pygeum africanum: 100 mg/day after food

Curcuma longa (bioavailable form): up to 8 g/day equiv. curcumin after food

Zingiber officinale: 1.2 g/day in dried root tablet/capsule with food

ESSIAC tea (proprietary blend containing: *Arctium lappa*, *Rheum* spp., *Rumex acetosella* and *Ulmus rubra*): 2 cups a day (5 g per cup)

Nutritional prescription

Co-Q10: 150 mg 2–3 × daily after food

Vitamin D3: 2000 IU/day with food

Melatonin: 5 mg at night before bed

Pomegranate juice: 230 mL/day

Lifestyle prescription

Moderate exercise

Good sleep hygiene and mindfulness meditation

Dietary improvement

- Omega-3 fatty acids are also advised via an increase of deep-sea oily fish and polyunsaturated-rich seeds in the diet, or via supplementation if required.

Expected outcomes and follow-up protocols

It is vital when treating a patient with prostate cancer to monitor compliance. In the abovementioned case, the dietary and lifestyle changes may be difficult to implement and adhere to for certain individuals. Their partner or friends may support them in implementing and sustaining the changes required. If the suggestions are adhered to, the patient should generally feel a lot better with increased energy, better quality sleep and minor weight loss within the first month. Withdrawal of alcohol and cigarettes may change this perception as the initial response of abstinence will make the patient feel worse before feeling better. After the second to third month of the program symptoms should be markedly improved.

Other modalities may assist in reducing cigarette and alcohol consumption such as acupuncture and/or hypnosis. Due to the patient's cardiovascular disease, seeing an exercise physiologist or certified personal trainer may assist with his exercise program. Ideally, after the 3 (preferably 6) months of natural therapy treatment, the PSA will hopefully have decreased and the two spots on the MRI should be stable. The patient can then choose what path to take next—either to choose a radical prostatectomy, radiation/brachytherapy, androgen-deprivation therapy or to continue on the natural therapy program for another 3–6 months and be monitored again after that period.

Clinical pearls

- When treating someone with prostate cancer, it is important to know their Gleason score more than their PSA level as research shows that the PSA can vary dramatically and not always be a good indicator of prostate cancer status.

- Always assess the patient's psychological state with the diagnosis of cancer.

- Always treat the individual first rather than the disease.

- Stage treatment rather than overwhelming the person with everything at once.

Expert | CONSULT

Clinical Comprehension Questions & Answers are hosted on
https://expertconsult.inkling.com/store/book/
sarris-clinical-naturopathy-case-files-1

BIBLIOGRAPHY

Chai W, Cooney RV, Franke AA, et al. Plasma coenzyme Q10 levels and prostate cancer risk: the multiethnic cohort study. *Cancer Epidemiol Biomarkers Prev*. 2011;20(4):708-710.

Hasenoehrl T, Keilani M, Komanadj T, et al (2015) 'The effects of resistance exercise on physical performance and health-related quality of life in prostate cancer patients: a systematic review.' *Support Care Cancer*. 2015;23(8):2479-2497.

Paller CJ, Ye X, Wozniak PJ, et al. A randomised phase II study of pomegranate extract for men with rising PSA following initial therapy for localized prostate cancer. *Prostate Cancer Prostatic Dis*. 2013;16(1):50-55.

Schloss J. Cancer. In: Sarris J, Wardle J, eds. *Clinical Naturopathy: An Evidence-Based Guide to Practice*. 2nd ed. Sydney: Elsevier; 2014.

Yang M, Kenfield SA, Van Blarigan EL, et al. Dietary patterns after prostate cancer diagnosis in relation to disease-specific and total mortality. *Cancer Prev Res (Phila)*. 2015;8(6):545-551.

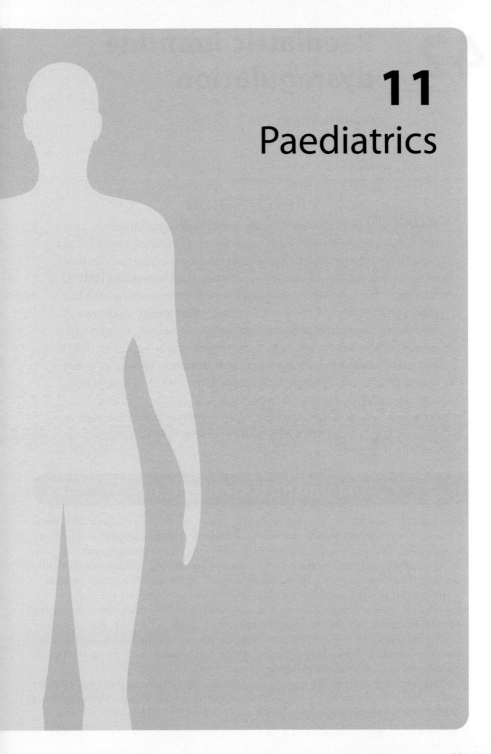

11
Paediatrics

42 Paediatric immune dysregulation

Diana Bowman

PRESENTATION

A **4-year-old girl** is brought to the clinic by her grandmother, who has a share of the primary care since the child's mother returned to work 9 months ago. The child is 'unable to attend school today due to yet another cold'. **Acute upper respiratory tract infections (URTIs)** have occurred every few months since beginning kindergarten last year. She typically presents with **runny, clear nasal discharge**, a **mild fever, headache** and **malaise**, which are usually treated with courses of antibiotics. She has trouble sleeping when she has a URTI and **wakes coughing** during the night. She often suffers an **upset stomach** with **wind pain and flatulence**. The child has always been a **'fussy' eater**, refusing to eat vegetables except for peas and deep-fried potatoes, and the only fruit eaten is canned with ice-cream or custard. She is a **sensitive, shy and reserved** child.

Diagnostic considerations

There are many reasons for lowered immunity including poor sleep, poor diet, stress or exposure to pollutants or cigarette smoke. Children's immune systems undergo vast changes in the first years of life and are extremely sensitive to endogenous and exogenous signalling. This makes them highly susceptible to viral illnesses, in particular respiratory tract infections, which, due to their viral origins, do not require antibiotics.

The highest priority in treating a case such as this is to address the acute symptoms. Reducing respiratory inflammation and curbing pathogenesis while supporting immune resistance are the main acute treatment aims. To reduce the chronicity of symptoms and additional bouts of illness, further treatment should concentrate on addressing the underlying, exacerbating imbalances such as psychological, physiological and gastrointestinal dysfunction.

Catarrhal congestion of the mucous membranes and resultant postnasal drip are most probably the causes of the night-time cough. This leads to poor sleep, but for a sensitive, shy child starting a new routine such as starting kindergarten, establishing friendships and spending time without mother can be extremely stressful, resulting in heightened anxiety that may be contributing to disturbed sleep patterns. The links between reduced immune function and gastrointestinal tract (GIT) dysregulation are well documented. Intestinal microflora imbalances are likely causes of the GIT discomfort and can promote further infections, forming a vicious cycle leading to a more permanent immune imbalance.

NATUROPATHIC TREATMENT AIMS IN PAEDIATRIC MANAGEMENT
- Treat acute symptoms
- Strengthen immune defences
- Correct digestive function
- Support the nervous system
- Support a healthy appetite and balanced diet

Treatment protocol

- Short-term immune, antiviral and anticatarrhal support is required for the symptomatic relief of respiratory conditions. The addition of anti-inflammatory and sedative herbs should begin to address the underlying GIT and nervous system dysregulation.
- *Echinacea* spp. is traditionally indicated for preventing and treating URTIs. The immunomodulator activity of *Echinacea* spp. has been the subject of numerous studies (some of which are not supportive). Clinical evidence for its inclusion in this formula is based mostly on positive results in adults with URTIs.
- *Pelargonium sidoides* is an immune-modulator, antiviral and antibacterial herbal medicine that has been investigated as a promising treatment for managing respiratory tract infections. It has shown an ability to mobilise natural killer cells to deal with invading pathogens. Antibacterial properties restrict bacteria from adhering to healthy mucosal cells, while its mucolytic properties stimulate respiratory cilia. This transports viscous mucus away therefore reducing bacteria numbers by removing the bacteria's nutrient base.
- *Sambucus nigra* (flower) has revealed evidence of antiviral, anti-inflammatory, antioxidant and antibacterial properties, while the berry has demonstrated antioxidant and antiviral activities.
- *Matricaria recutita* is used due to its sedative and carminative properties and is well indicated for children with nervous system and GIT challenges.
- Probiotics increase the proliferation of beneficial intestinal microbiota and strengthen the intestinal barrier. Probiotics containing *Lactobacillus rhamnosus* GG, *Streptococcus thermophiles*, *Lactobacillus acidophilus* and *Bifidobacterium* spp. have the potential to enhance immune function and

have a demonstrated an ability to diminish the incidence of infection and/or curtail infection duration. A wide range of dosages (100 million to 1.8 trillion colony-forming units (CFUs) per day) have been studied in clinical trials. Generally, higher dosages of probiotics (> 5 billion CFUs/day in children) were associated with more significant results. Choose a probiotic specifically formulated for children and follow the manufacturer's recommendations for dosages.

- Vitamin C is considered crucial for children's health and development and is often found to be deficient in children with poor appetites and who are finicky about food choices. Vitamin C is water-soluble and, while intake is best from food sources, the recommended supplementation is 35 mg/day. However, vitamin C treatment of URTIs for 4–8-year-old children can be increased to 600–1000 mg per day. Vitamin C is best given in divided doses with food throughout the day.

- Zinc is used in more than 200 enzyme pathways in the body and is essential for growth and development as well as normal immune responses. Immune deficiencies increase the need for zinc, and a low-protein diet is a common cause of zinc deficiency. Zinc supplementation is indicated in chronic infections, and zinc picolinate is better absorbed than other forms. The recommended intake for zinc is 4–12 mg/day for 4–8-year-old children. The adult dose of zinc picolinate is 30–60 mg per day (use Clark's

PRESCRIPTION
Herbal formula (100 mL)

Echinacea spp. 1:2	30 mL
Pelargonium sidoides 1:2	25 mL
Matricaria recutita 1:2	25 mL
Sambucus nigra 1:2	20 mL

Dose: (Young's rule) 1.25 mL 3 × daily before meals

Nutritional prescription

Vitamin C: 600 mg/day (200 mg 3 × daily with food) until food sources improve

Child-specific probiotic supplement: dosage as per manufacturer's recommendation

Lifestyle prescription

Introduce vitamin C food sources to the daily diet: oranges, grapefruit, red and green capsicum, kiwifruit, broccoli, strawberries, cantaloupe, baked potatoes and tomatoes

Probiotic foods include artichokes, garlic, onion, leeks, asparagus, chives, legumes, peas and fruit—many of these may be disguised in other dishes, such as soups and casseroles rule to calculate the correct dosage). Zinc may be better tolerated when given at night.

Expected outcomes and follow-up protocols

The best outcomes come from the child, parents and practitioner working together. The highest priority in treating a case such as this is to address the acute symptoms. Reducing respiratory inflammation and curbing pathogenesis while supporting immune resistance are the main acute treatment aims. To reduce chronicity of symptoms and additional bouts of illness, further treatment should concentrate on addressing the underlying, exacerbating imbalances such as psychological, physiological and gastrointestinal dysfunction. Aiming for achievable goals will lessen frustrations.

Frequent follow-ups are important, with emotional support for both the parents and the child, and to ensure the educative approach to treatment. Frequent follow-ups are also important because paediatric conditions can change significantly in a short period of time, and any medications should be given only where necessary, as infrequently as possible, and monitored with caution.

Treatment should focus on acute symptoms as they arise. Unlike adults, children are growing and developing, so it is best to focus any long-term treatment on diet and lifestyle factors that facilitate healthy growth and development, rather than trying to medicate them. If there are underlying immunological issues, investigate underlying

CALCULATING CHILDREN'S DOSES OF SPECIFIC TREATMENTS

The correct dosage for children is simply achieved by choosing the most appropriate calculation.

HERBAL MEDICINES

1. Ausberger's rule (based on weight): $(1.5 \times \text{weight in kg}) + 10 = \%$ adult dose

2. Clark's rule (based on weight): $\dfrac{\text{Weight in kg} \times \text{adult dose}}{67} = \text{child's dose}$

3. Young's rule (based on age): $\dfrac{\text{Age in years} \times \text{adult dose}}{(\text{age} + 12)} = \text{child's dose}$

4. Fried's rule (best for infants): $\dfrac{\text{Age in months} \times \text{adult dose}}{150} = \text{child's dose}$

NUTRIENTS

Age-related nutritional requirements are found within the government guidelines for recommended daily intake (RDI). Dosage for nutritional medicines with adult-only recommendations may be calculated using Clark's rule. Extemporaneous dispensing of specific nutrients may be calculated at mg/kg of body weight for children's dosages.

causes such as healthy microbiome, food sensitivities or emotional distress rather than developing a reliance on long-term use of supplements.

Clinical pearls

- Education, explanation and motivation through positive feedback develop the basis of treatment in paediatric care.

- Address the underlying, exacerbating imbalances that create recurrent illnesses.

- Use age-appropriate dosages of herbs, supplements and medicinal foods.

- Probiotics may cause bloating if used in a high dosage.

- Small, well-aimed prescriptions present best practice with minimum intervention and maximum result.

Expert | CONSULT

Clinical Comprehension Questions & Answers are hosted on
**https://expertconsult.inkling.com/store/book/
sarris-clinical-naturopathy-case-files-1**

BIBLIOGRAPHY

Casteleijn D, Finney-Brown T. Respiratory infections and immune deficiency. In: Sarris J, Wardle J, eds. *Clinical Naturopathy: An Evidence-Based Guide to Practice.* 2nd ed. Sydney: Elsevier; 2014.

Hunt K, Ernst E. The evidence-base for complementary medicine in children: a critical overview of systematic reviews. *Arch Dis Child.* 2011;96(8):769-776.

Mortimer V. Paediatrics. In: Sarris J, Wardle J, eds. *Clinical Naturopathy: An Evidence-Based Guide to Practice.* 2nd ed. Sydney: Elsevier; 2014.

Marques AH, O'Connor TG, Roth C, et al. The influence of maternal prenatal and early childhood nutrition and maternal prenatal stress on offspring immune system development and neurodevelopmental disorders. *Front Neurosci.* 2013;7:120.

Santich R, Bone K. *Phytotherapy Essentials: Healthy Children: Optimising Children's Health With Herbs.* Warwick: Phytotherapy Press; 2008.

United Nations. Conventions on the Rights of the Child. General Assembly resolution 44/25 of 20 November 1989 Geneva, Switzerland: Online. Available: http://www.unicef.org/crc.1989 1 Nov 2013.

43 Nocturnal enuresis

Diana Bowman

PRESENTATION

A **7-year-old boy** who has recently moved house with his parents to a new area and a new school **presents with bedwetting**. He has been typically quite well, is current with all childhood vaccinations (to which he had no serious reactions) and is a little **inclined to anxiety** at times of change or stress in the family. He **presents with feeling upset in his stomach** and **not wanting to eat, constipation** and a **history of bedwetting** since the family moved house (he had stopped wetting the bed a year ago at the age of 6). He has experienced an **increase in crying episodes** and not wanting to meet new friends at school or play with other children after school.

Diagnostic considerations

Secondary nocturnal enuresis (SNE) is diagnosed in children who have had a period of dryness of more than 6 months and enuresis has started again. The main aim in treating the above case is to find and ameliorate the underlying cause, which can prove difficult with a child who is already anxious and withdrawn. To gain the child's trust, a practitioner must pay particular attention to conveying a sense of compassion and understanding, not only to the child but to the parents as well. The child must feel safe to share their secret and be confident there will be no judgement or recriminations.

The constipation in this case could be a complicating and/or causative factor in the SNE. It is most likely contributing to the upset stomach and poor appetite and may have been the chief cause of the gastrointestinal tract disturbances initially. An altered appetite may exacerbate constipation and anxiety due to a diet low in fibre and nutrients such as magnesium.

For a sensitive child, settling into a new area and school and finding new friends can be extremely stressful, resulting in social withdrawal and heightened anxiety, which may be contributing to the stomach upset with concomitant poor appetite and constipation. The goal is for a happy, confident child who enjoys dry nights, restful sleep and the company of his peers. It may be useful to refer him to a medical doctor or specialist clinic to exclude organic causative factors or to seek professional counselling if the child has difficulty discussing their concerns with his parents or practitioner.

NATUROPATHIC TREATMENT AIMS IN NERVOUS SYSTEM CONDITIONS IN CHILDREN

- Discover and treat the cause(s) to provide relief to the child and family
- Calm the nervous system and support psychologically
- Support a healthy appetite and normal bowel motions
- Provide a plan to reduce the recurrence of the disorder after treatment ceases

Treatment protocol

- Mostly, nocturnal enuresis does not require medication; however, short-term herbal medication may assist in comorbid conditions such as anxiety and constipation. Resolving these issues is paramount to treatment, particularly if they are causative factors.

- *Passiflora incarnata* has anxiolytic and sedative activity and is a popular herb for nervousness and anxiety. Traditionally used for various nervous system disorders, recent evidence has shown the herb's anxiolytic effects are mediated via the GABAergic system. Some practitioners have reservations about prescribing mild hypnotics during the day; however, clinical evidence has confirmed no effect on job performance compared with benzodiazepines.

- *Turnera diffusa* acts as a nervine tonic, tonic and mild laxative. Its potential indications include anxiety, depression, nervous dyspepsia and constipation.

- *Matricaria recutita* is a mild sedative and carminative. It is often prescribed safely to children for upset stomach and anxiety conditions.

- *Glycyrrhiza glabra* is indicated for treating constipation and, as a traditional 'adrenal tonic', may assist in alleviating the long-term, underlying effects of anxiety.

- Where there is a nutritional deficiency, supplements can be useful. Selenium may be indicated—low dietary selenium has been associated with a number of cases of anxiety, depression and tiredness. A word of caution about prescribing selenium for children: Always confirm a deficiency exists and never exceed the recommended dose (see prescription box).

- Dietary advice is fundamental to success in this case. Foods rich in magnesium, calcium and zinc provide the building blocks for healthy growth and maturation for cells and metabolic pathways. Assessment for allergies/intolerances, minimising nutrient-deficient food choices and teaching good dietary habits is imperative.

- Other integrative medical therapies have proven useful. Hypnotherapy and guided imagery can show good results for children with SNE. Acupuncture has demonstrated effectiveness for treating nocturnal enuresis.

PRESCRIPTION
Herbal formula (100 mL)

Passiflora incarnata 1:2	30 mL
Turnera diffusa 1:2	25 mL
Matricaria recutita 1:2	25 mL
Glycyrrhiza glabra 1:1	20 mL

Dose: (Young's rule) 2 mL 3 × daily after meals

Nutritional prescription

Selenium: 30 mcg/day for 5 weeks

Lifestyle prescription

Aim to achieve sufficient magnesium, calcium and zinc in the diet via almonds, cashews, cocoa, molasses, parsnips, soya beans, wholegrain cereals, meat, fish, yoghurt and bok choi

Expected outcomes and follow-up protocols

A cohesive partnership between the child, his parents and his practitioner will see the best results. Resolution may be expected within a few months, provided there is compliance to treatment. Understanding both the child's and the parents' perceptions will help in creating a manageable treatment plan with achievable goals that encourage self-esteem and diminish frustrations. The child needs to be completely engaged in the treatment process in order to feel they have contributed to it. Frequent follow-ups are important to continue the emotional support and encouragement for the parents and child. Repeated wet nights are common at the beginning of treatment, along with the occasional setback, but relying on positive feedback and small rewards (not focusing on negative outcomes) helps to motivate and educate the family while the treatment goals are being met.

Meditation and relaxation techniques encourage composure and self-concept and are enjoyable pursuits for children, which will be useful during the treatment and may also help to maintain the dry state after treatments have ceased. With a supportive familial environment and the anxiety managed, SNE should resolve quite quickly, with the child experiencing dry nights every night within 2–3 months. At the resolution of the condition herbal and supplement treatment may be discontinued; however, the dietary considerations should remain in place to ensure complete nutrition to support healthy nervous, digestive and immune function.

Clinical pearls

- Education, explanation and motivation through positive feedback develop the basis of treatment.

- Parents, the patient and siblings all require support and some treatment.

- Encourage healthy attitudes to digestion and elimination in the early years to promote lifelong health.

- Always investigate potential organic causes of the condition and eliminate food intolerances or allergies as causative agents.

Expert | CONSULT

Clinical Comprehension Questions & Answers are hosted on **https://expertconsult.inkling.com/store/book/ sarris-clinical-naturopathy-case-files-1**

BIBLIOGRAPHY

Glazner C, Evans J, Cheuk D. Complementary and miscellaneous interventions for nocturnal enuresis in children. *Cochrane Database Syst Rev.* 2005;(2):CD005230.

Hunt K, Ernst E. The evidence base for complementary medicine in children: a critical overview of systematic reviews. *Arch Dis Child.* 2011;96(8):769-776.

Mortimer V. Paediatrics. In: Sarris J, Wardle J, eds. *Clinical Naturopathy: An Evidence-Based Guide to Practice.* ed 2. Sydney: Elsevier; 2014.

Santich R, Bone K. *Phytotherapy Essentials: Healthy Children: Optimising Children's Health With Herbs.* Warwick: Phytotherapy Press; 2008.

United Nations. Conventions on the Rights of the Child. General Assembly resolution 44/25 of 20 November 1989 Geneva, Switzerland: Online. Available: http://www.unicef.org/crc.1989 1 Nov 2013.

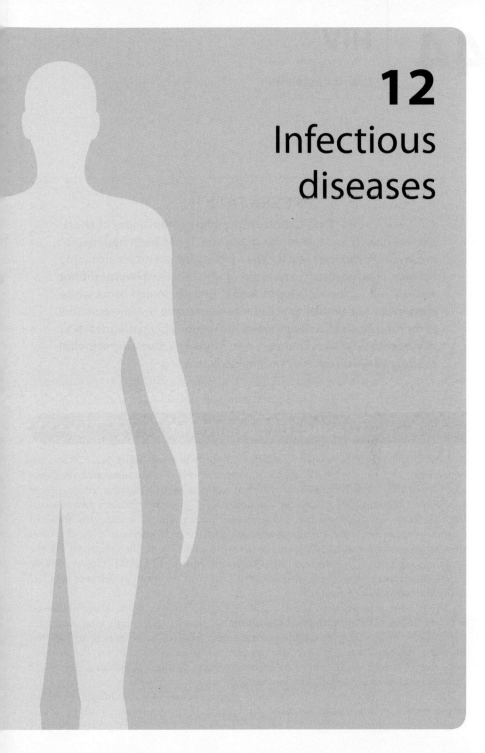

12
Infectious diseases

44 HIV

David Casteleijn

PRESENTATION

A 34-year-old woman presents to the clinic complaining of **shortness of breath** and a **chronic cough**, which has been getting progressively worse over the past 3 years. She has also noted increasing **fatigue** for no apparent reason, along with recurrent **overnight hot flushes** and increasingly **loose stools**. She has noted some **white plaques in her mouth**, which she assumed was thrush secondary to recent courses of antibiotics. She has recently been **diagnosed as HIV positive** and been commenced on **highly active antiretroviral therapy (HAART)** because her viral load was high.

Diagnostic considerations

Because it is possible to remain relatively symptom-free for many years after seroconversion, the time between the production of HIV antibodies and diagnosis can vary widely. This dictates very different courses of naturopathic treatment. It is relatively common for people who acquire HIV infection through heterosexual intercourse to be diagnosed late in the course of the illness, leading the focus of treatment to be both the current symptoms and the side effects of HAART once that has been commenced. With this patient the majority of her symptoms are the result of long-term HIV infection rather than side effects of HAART. However, these potential adverse effects should still be taken into consideration, as this will help her maintain continuity of treatment.

The patient presents with chronic diarrhoea and fatigue, both of which can be a symptom of HIV progression or attributable to HAART. High viral loads are particularly associated with fatigue, as the body requires more energy to fuel the immune response. Fatigue may also be due to vitamin or mineral deficiencies, poor sleep, anxiety, depression or other concomitant medical conditions. The white plaques, night sweats and shortness of breath are all symptoms of later-stage HIV and dropping CD4 counts. White plaques may represent oral candidiasis (in which case they will be removable) or hairy leukoplakia (non-removable), both of which become more common as the CD4 count falls. Around half of HIV-positive patients experience night sweats not related to exercise or room temperature, and these can be profuse and disruptive. Shortness of breath (dyspnoea) may be attributable to infective causes (usually associated with cough and fever) or non-infective causes such as anaemia, asthma, heart failure or Kaposi's sarcoma in the lungs. It is important to differentiate between causes of dyspnoea, as these will require different treatments. Patients with pneumonia require antibiotic treatment.

The patient is undertaking an effective conventional treatment (HAART) that aims to reduce the viral load to undetectable levels and keep it there. It is important to educate the patient that herbal and nutritional support for her condition is *not* intended to replace HAART, and that she should continue with her medications. Sporadic adherence to these is associated with drug resistance.

SUGGESTIVE SYMPTOMS IN HIV PATIENTS
- Persistent cough
- Shortness of breath
- Soaking night sweats
- Gastrointestinal tract disturbance
- Chronic diarrhoea
- White spots on the tongue and mouth
- Weight loss

Treatment protocol

- *Echinacea* spp. has immune-enhancing and immune-modulating properties. Extracts of *Echinacea purpurea* have shown the ability to stimulate cellular immune function in vitro in patients with AIDS. The root blend is superior in this case as the alkylamides in *Echinacea purpurea* appear to enhance the action of those in *Echinacea angustifolia,* therefore enhancing their effect. Late last century, a theoretical concern was raised about stimulating the immune system and therefore increasing viral load. However, multiple studies from 2010 onwards have shown that co-administration of *Echinacea purpurea* and the HAART medications lopinavir, etravirine, darunavir and ritonavir in HIV-infected patients is safe and well tolerated, with no effect on drug pharmacokinetics and no increase in viral load.

- *Hydrastis canadensis* is considered to be a mucous membrane trophorestorative and in practice provides significant relief from the gastrointestinal tract disturbance commonly found in HIV infection. This includes both the diarrhoea and any oral thrush. As the actives are alkaloids, care should be taken not to use high-tannin herbs because the alkaloids will bind with the tannins and may not cleave off during transit through the digestive tract, potentially being wasted.

- *Withania somnifera* and *Astragalus membranaceus* are adaptogens and general tonics that help with energy and vitality and support the immune system.

- *Curcuma longa* is anti-inflammatory, antioxidant, hypolipidaemic, anti-microbial and carminative, which are all important actions in supporting HIV. Initially the liquid is prescribed as part of the mixture because direct contact with the digestive tract is desired. As treatment progresses this may be exchanged for a curcuma/phospholipid complex that has demonstrated a sound absorption profile.

- A plant-based 'gastrointestinal powder' formula is prescribed—there are many different versions of this available, but the key ingredients are glutamine and sources of soluble fibres such as *Ulmus rubra* and *Actinidia deliciosa*.

- All herbal medicines should be given away from HAART medications to reduce the risk of lowering drug absorption from the gastrointestinal tract.

- In addition, care must be taken when prescribing herbs or nutrients that may strongly stimulate liver detoxification pathways, as these may change the pharmacokinetics of conventional medicines.

- Consider specific nutrient therapy to address any particular vitamin or mineral deficiencies identified by pathology testing and dietary recall (i.e. iron/B12 for anaemia).

- Vegetable broths, bean and vegetable stews, rice congee and homemade chicken soup (with the whole carcass from organic chicken) provide essential immune-supportive nutrients. The importance of colour variety is stressed as this broadens the range of nutrients ingested.

- Patients with HIV are more at risk of foodborne infections and so should ideally avoid unpasteurised dairy, raw eggs and raw seafood.

- Daily exercise without overexertion is important from both a physical and psychological perspective.

- Yoga and meditation may be helpful for emotional health, helping to reduce levels of stress and anxiety. There is some evidence that mindfulness meditation may buffer CD4+ T-lymphocyte count, which declines in those with HIV.

Expected outcomes and follow-up protocols

Initially, the clinician should assess if any general quality of life improvements are occurring, with enhanced overall vitality and decreased fatigue being demonstrated. This should be evident in the first couple of weeks with the above treatment, but it is

PRESCRIPTION
Herbal formula (100 mL)

Astragalus membranaceus 1:2	30 mL
Echinacea spp. root blend (60/40 *E. purpurea/E. angustifolia*) 1:2	20 mL
Curcuma longa 1:1	20 mL
Hydrastis canadensis 1:3	15 mL
Withania somnifera 2:1	15 mL

Dose: 5 mL 3 × daily in a little water or juice

Nutritional prescription

Glutamine insoluble fibre combination: 1 tsp in 200 mL of water or juice morning and night

Lifestyle prescription

Graded exercise and yoga

vital to remain alert for side effects of HAART or other difficulties over the long term. With improvements in therapies it is now possible for a person who is HIV positive but well managed on HAART (i.e. undetectable viral load) to have a life expectancy very similar to that which they would have had if they were not HIV positive.

Although this trend is not necessarily found in all people who are HIV positive, it is a good incentive for your patient to remain on HAART and to encourage them to discuss their side effects with you and their medical practitioner to find a way of mitigating these and assisting long-term compliance with the HAART regimen. It is now recommended that all people with HIV consider starting HAART, irrespective of how long the person has been HIV positive or what their viral load or CD4 count is. Not only is this considered to reduce the health problems associated with HIV (cardiovascular disease, cancers, bone disorders and cognitive problems) but also reduces the risk of transmitting HIV (in association with standard infection control measures such as condoms and sterile injecting equipment).

Clinical pearls

- With good outcomes evident from HAART, every effort should be taken to help the patient maintain their prescribed regimen.

- It is not always possible to discern whether HIV progression or HAART therapy has caused a particular symptom. However, regardless of the cause, symptom reduction or resolution (where possible) will improve quality of life.

- Natural medicine is not an alternative to conventional therapies, nor a cure for HIV, but may provide great improvements in quality of life, which should always be the end goal for the practitioner.

Expert | CONSULT

Clinical Comprehension Questions & Answers are hosted on
https://expertconsult.inkling.com/store/book/
sarris-clinical-naturopathy-case-files-1

BIBLIOGRAPHY

Creswell J, Myers HF, Cole SW, et al. Mindfulness meditation training effects on CD4+ T lymphocytes in HIV-1 infected adults: a small randomized controlled trial. *Brain Behav Immun.* 2009;23(2):184-188.

Hillier J. Human immunodeficiency virus. In: Sarris J, Wardle J, eds. *Clinical Naturopathy: An Evidence-Based Guide to Practice.* Sydney: Elsevier; 2014.

May M, Gompels M, Sabin C. Abstracts of the Eleventh International Congress on Drug Therapy in HIV Infection. *J Int AIDS Soc.* 2012;15(suppl 4):18078.

Molto J, Valle M, Miranda C, et al. Herb–drug interaction between *Echinacea purpurea* and Darunavir-Ritonavir in HIV-infected patients. *Antimicrob Agents Chemother.* 2011;55(1):326-330.

Penzac SR, Robertson SM, Hunt JD, et al. *Echinacea purpurea* significantly induces cytochrome P450 3A (CYP3A) but does not alter Lopinavir-Ritonavir exposure in healthy subjects. *Pharmacother.* 2010;30(8):797-805.

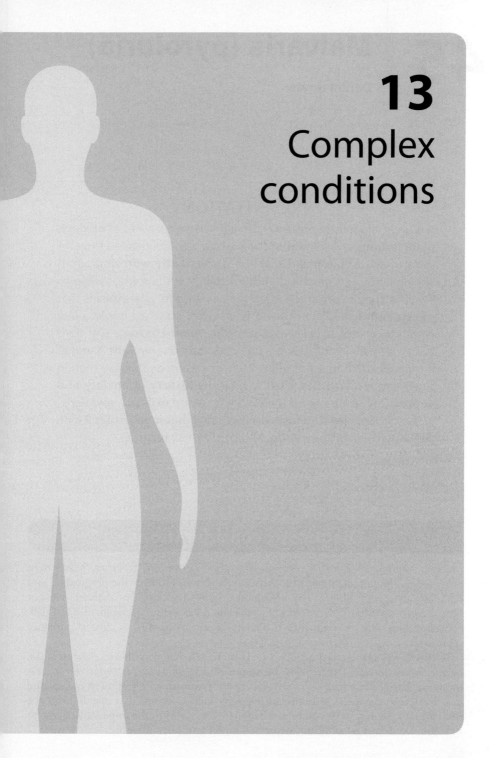

13
Complex conditions

45

Malvaria (pyroluria)

Daniel Roytas

PRESENTATION

A 20-year-old female presents with a primary complaint of **anxiety**, **mood swings** and **irritability**, which she has experienced since 14 years of age. She explains that she is **constantly worrying** about 'the smallest and most insignificant things', finds it impossible to 'switch her mind off' and has a 'negative attitude'. She explains that she **craves alcohol**, consuming four or five standard drinks every night to be able to relax and stop the **'mind chatter'**. She does not participate in any exercise and is **slightly overweight**. Her diet is primarily comprised of refined, processed foods that are high in sugar and saturated fat. There is a **family history of anxiety and depression**. A functional pathology test for malvaria (pyroluria) indicated an **elevated urinary hydroxyl haemopyrrolin-2-one (HPL) pyrrole concentration** 48 mcg/dL (0–20 mcg/dL).

Diagnostic considerations

Malvaria (pyroluria) is not a recognised medical condition; however, it has been proposed as a potentially useful biochemical marker to monitor the progression and remission of mental illness. The biological origins and causes of malvaria are not completely understood, therefore clinicians should interpret elevated urinary HPL concentrations with caution until further evidence to support its clinical relevance is available.

Elevated urinary concentrations of HPL are associated with zinc, magnesium, niacin and pyridoxine deficiencies. Deficiencies of these nutrients negatively impact on the synthesis and activity of a range of neurotransmitters, resulting in mental and emotional disturbances. Other presenting signs and symptoms that may indicate the need for an HPL test to be conducted include white flecks in the fingernails, frequent infections, anaemia, alcoholism, depressed mood and poor memory.

Common theorised causes of elevated urinary HPL concentrations include altered haem breakdown and synthesis, dietary intake, intestinal dysbiosis, heavy metal toxicity, allergy, oxidative stress, adrenal fatigue and genetic disorders. Due to the wide range of potential contributing factors, a thorough case history and physical examination should be undertaken to elucidate the underlying cause. Pathology tests such as haemoglobin, blood histamine, homocysteine, hair mineral analysis, salivary cortisol, porphyrins and a digestive stool analysis may be necessary to confirm the differential diagnosis.

Due to the family history of anxiety and depression, the patient may have inherited a genetic predisposition that results in altered haemoglobin synthesis and subsequent elevations in HPL. A nutritional genetic profile may be warranted to identify single nucleotide polymorphisms contributing to the patient's symptoms. MTHFR C677T and 1298C mutations are commonly associated with elevated HPL concentrations, which negatively impact on methylation pathways as well as red blood cell synthesis and function.

MEDICAL CONDITIONS THAT MAY PRESENT WITH HIGH MALVARIA

- Autism
- Attention deficit disorder (ADD) or attention deficit and hyperactivity disorder (ADHD)
- Hyperhomocysteinaemia
- Anaemia
- Irritable bowel syndrome or dysbiosis
- Single nucleotide polymorphisms (SNPs) of methylation genes
- Anxiety
- Depression
- Adrenal insufficiency
- Substance abuse
- Hypoglycaemia

Treatment protocol

- Due to the potential deficiencies of pyridoxine, magnesium, niacin and zinc, supplementation of these nutrients can be considered as a potential first-line therapy. Supplementation should begin immediately, with the aim of reducing the symptoms of anxiety, mood swings, irritability and alcohol cravings. Once supplementation has begun, further testing can then be undertaken to identify and treat the underlying cause.

- Zinc supplementation is prescribed to address the potential deficiency associated with malvaria. Deficiencies in zinc can cause altered brain function because it is required for the storage of histamine within the hippocampus to facilitate histaminergic neurotransmission, cellular serotonin uptake and modulation of the N-methyl-D-aspartate (NMDA)/glutamate pathway.

- Magnesium plays an integral role in regulating neuronal nitric oxide production and may elicit an anxiolytic activity through its involvement in the NMDA/glutamate pathway. Magnesium deficiency can lead to impaired neurotransmission of serotonergic, cholinergic and noradrenergic structures, giving rise to mental and emotional disturbances.

- Vitamin B6 supplementation reduces urinary zinc excretion. B6 is also integral for the production of several hormones including serotonin and noradrenaline. Patients with compromised methylation also require pyridoxine supplementation to support homocysteine metabolism.

- Patients identified with MTHFR C677T and 1298C mutations may require additional supplementation of B2, B3, B9 and B12 to overcome impaired homocysteine metabolism and other methylation-dependent processes.

- *Silybum marianum* is advised to counteract the burden placed on the liver with excessive alcohol intake due to its hepatoprotective and hepatic trophorestorative effects.

- Dietary modification should include increased intake of green leafy vegetables, fruits, whole grains, nuts and seeds coupled with a reduced intake of alcohol, confectionery and processed/refined foods. An exercise program promoting cardiovascular health and weight loss may also be beneficial for this patient.

- Chelation therapy (if needed) is recommended for patients with heavy metal toxicity, which can be facilitated through additional supplementation of vitamin C, manganese, selenium and N-acetylcysteine and increased dietary fibre intake.

PRESCRIPTION
Herbal formula

Silybum marianum capsules equivalent to 140 mg of flavonolignans
Dose: 1 capsule 3 × daily

Nutritional prescription

Zinc citrate: 1 tablet (20 mg elemental) 3 × daily after food
Magnesium amino acid chelate: 2 tablets (80 mg elemental) 2 × daily after food
Pyridoxal-5-phosphate: 2 capsules (50 mg) 2 × daily after food
Methylcobalamin 5000 mcg chewable tablet: 1 tablet daily after food

Lifestyle prescription

Increase fruit intake to two serves 5 × per week and vegetable intake to five serves per day
30 minutes or more of moderate exercise per day (brisk walking/yoga)
Mindfulness/meditation for 10–15 minutes per day
Reduce alcohol consumption

Expected outcomes and follow-up protocols

The proposed treatment is expected to decrease HPL concentrations; however, it is important for clinicians to remember that this test is not diagnostic and that elevated HPL is not a medical condition. It is expected that, if this is the correct approach for this patient (taking into consideration other unknown factors), noticeable changes in the patient's mood will occur within 7 days of beginning treatment. Practitioners should schedule a follow-up appointment within 7 days of the initial treatment to monitor patient compliance and tolerance to treatment.

Supplementation of B6, zinc, niacin and magnesium can continue until other underlying causes have been identified and treated appropriately. For example, patients with malvaria caused by intestinal permeability are unlikely to require ongoing nutritional supplementation once normal gut function has been restored. Conversely, patients with malvaria caused by a genetic disorder may require supplementation indefinitely. The patient should be retested for HPL at 12 weeks to gauge the efficacy of treatment and dosage modifications implemented where necessary.

The patient should be monitored for signs of B6 and zinc toxicity due to the high-dose prescription. Within 7 days of B6 supplementation, improved sleep duration and quality is expected; however, reports of excessive dreaming may indicate the dose of B6 is too high. Long-term B6 toxicity can result in peripheral neuropathy (tingling in the toes); however, the use of pyridoxal-5-phosphate (P5P) may be able to reduce this risk. Once the deficiency has been addressed, the prescription should be revised and dosages modified to maintain normal levels of these nutrients.

In summary, it should be noted that it is unknown from an evidentiary perspective whether this nutrient supplement approach will ameliorate her symptoms. However, as there is no medical diagnosis for her symptoms and the treatment approach is inexpensive, such a therapeutic approach may be beneficial.

Clinical pearls

- Elevated blood histamine levels may be indicative of under-methylation while low levels indicate over-methylation.

- A copper:zinc ratio of approximately 2:1 is common in patients with a zinc deficiency and suffering from malvaria. Zinc supplementation should be aimed at achieving an optimal red blood cell copper:zinc ratio of 1:1.

- Up to 3000 mg per day of B6 has been used to treat patients with schizophrenia and malvaria, who may have HPL concentrations in excess of 350 mcg/dL.

- Use caution when prescribing higher doses of zinc (> 100 mg per day) because some patients may experience nausea.

Expert | CONSULT

Clinical Comprehension Questions & Answers are hosted on **https://expertconsult.inkling.com/store/book/ sarris-clinical-naturopathy-case-files-1**

BIBLIOGRAPHY

Jackson J, Braud M, Neathery S. Urine pyrroles and other orthomolecular tests in patients with ADD/ADHD. *J Orthomol Med.* 2010;25(1):39-42.

Jackson J, Riordan H, Neathery S, et al. Urinary pyrrole in health and disease. *J Orthomol Med.* 1997;12(2):96-98.

Mikirova N. Clinical test of pyrroles in psychiatric disorders: association with nutritional, immunological and metabolic markers. *J Nutr Ther.* 2015;4:4-11.

Mikirova N. Clinical test of pyrroles: usefulness and association with other biochemical markers. *Clin Med Rev Rep.* 2015;2(2):1-6.

Sarris J. Naturopathic diagnostic techniques. In: Sarris J, Wardle J, eds. *Clinical Naturopathy: An Evidence-Based Guide to Practice.* 2nd ed. Sydney: Elsevier; 2014.

46

Pain management

Justin Sinclair

PRESENTATION

A 69-year-old Caucasian male presented 2 months ago with **dull, burning pain and numbness in his right deltoid and trapezius** for a period of 10 days, which became associated with **unilaterally grouped erythematous vesicles** showing dermatomal distribution. Diagnosed with **herpes zoster**, his medical practitioner prescribed valacyclovir and paracetamol with codeine phosphate. Pain is still apparent after 2 months and the diagnosis of **post-herpetic neuralgia** was recently made. The patient is also **feeling anxious** and is experiencing bouts of **lower abdominal pain** and **diarrhoea** from his previously managed **irritable bowel syndrome**.

Diagnostic considerations

Pain is a disagreeable subjective physiological and psychosocial experience that often serves a biological purpose (warning of injury). It incorporates both the perception of a painful stimulus and the response to the perception. Physiologically, it can be classified into either of somatogenic (organic) or psychogenic (non-organic) origin. Somatogenic pain occurs as a result of a direct physiological mechanism or insult (such as osteoarthritis) and can be further divided into nociceptive pain (for example, ongoing activation of visceral nociceptors) or neuropathic pain (neurological dysfunction such as nerve compression). Pain can further be explained by duration of effect, being either acute (lasting less than 4 weeks) or chronic (lasting longer than 12 weeks).

Further compounding the deleterious physiological effects of pain are social, emotional and psychological ramifications, which are especially prevalent in chronic pain, causing debilitating sequelae such as affective disorders and comorbid depression. These cannot be ignored in differential diagnosis or in treatment. Factors such as age, gender, race and socioeconomic status are also important to consider in pain perception. Pain sufferers are often impaired in their ability to initiate or maintain fundamental daily activities such as eating, shopping and cleaning, further isolating the patient and increasing morbidity scales (decreasing quality of life).

Medical supervision and monitoring is strongly advised alongside concurrent complementary treatment to ensure analgesia is optimised. An integrative approach is considered best practice, as neuropathic pain can be difficult to manage. The flare up of irritable bowel syndrome (IBS) symptoms is most likely linked to his recent diagnosis, anxiety and prolonged pain, therefore focusing on pain management with symptomatic amelioration of anxiety and gastrointestinal tract issues is important in the initial stages. The patient should also be monitored for signs of depression, which is very common in postherpetic neuralgia (PHN).

COMMON CONDITIONS MANIFESTING PAIN

- Physiological (e.g. nociceptive acute trauma including either visceral, superficial or deep somatic pain)
- Chronic musculoskeletal (e.g. osteoarthritis, lumbago)
- Headaches (e.g. migraines, tension and cluster headaches)
- Nerve pain (e.g. herpes zoster, PHN)
- Cancer—pain can be due to either the disease itself (i.e. the tumour affecting surrounding tissues) or potential treatment such as surgery or radiotherapy
- Phantom pain (a form of neuropathic pain)
- Psychosomatic pain (i.e. psychogenic cause)

Treatment protocol

- A primary approach is to control pain with topical capsaicin cream (Zostrix 0.025% w/w) applied up to four times daily to the painful area. This should not be applied to broken skin. If the analgesic effect is insufficient, the topical capsaicin cream could be increased to 0.075% capsaicin concentration (Zostrix-HP). *Corydalis ambigua* can be used as needed for added analgesic support.

- Decreasing the viral load with antiviral herbs such as *Hypericum perforatum* (high hypericin concentration) or *Melissa officinalis* is important. If using *Hypericum* as an antiviral, choosing preparations that have low hyperforin concentration is imperative to reduce potential for interactions, which is likely with certain pharmaceuticals that may be used to manage this condition. Infused oil of *Hypericum* is also useful topically and may be considered as part of a management plan.

- Immune modulators/stimulants may provide assistance by preventing reactivation of the latent virus.

- Support the nervous system with nervine tonics and adaptogenic herbs.

- Symptomatic relief of comorbid anxiety is needed with anxiolytic herbs.

- Prescribe carminative and spasmolytic herbs to address the IBS symptomatology.

- Topical application of *Mentha x piperita* volatile oil (up to 10% menthol) has been shown in studies to provide relief to patients with PHN who were non-responsive to standard conventional treatments.

- Bulk demulcents such as *Ulmus rubra* and *Plantago psyllium* may be required to attenuate the diarrhoea. Physicochemical interactions need to be considered with coadministration of nutrients or herbal medicines.

- Eating a nutrient-dense diet is of great therapeutic value. Foods rich in B vitamins, taurine, serine, biotin, lipoic acid and copper may be of use in pain associated with nerve involvement.

- Gentle exercise like yoga and tai chi have been shown to improve anxiety. Mindfulness meditation and deep breathing exercises also have their place in assisting patients with chronic pain.

- Referring the patient to pain support groups or specialist pain clinics may be required.

PRESCRIPTION
Herbal formula 1 (100 mL)

Echinacea purpurea 1:2	25 mL
Passiflora incarnata 1:2	25 mL
Eleutherococcus senticosus 1:2	30 mL
Melissa officinalis 1:2	20 mL

Dose: 7.5 mL 2 × daily between meals

Herbal formula 2

Corydalis ambigua 1:2: 200 mL
Dose: 5–10 mL per day as needed for pain relief (tolerance can be developed)
Iberogast: 1 mL 3 × daily before meals
Zostrix 0.025% w/w capsaicin cream applied 3–4 × daily to the affected area. If non-responsive after 2 weeks, increase to Zostrix-HP (0.075% capsaicin)

Nutritional prescription

Vitamin C: 1000 mg up to 3 × daily
1 × B-complex tablet daily (morning)

Lifestyle prescription

Mindfulness meditation
Dietary improvement

Expected outcomes and follow-up protocols

Typically, pain relief from capsaicin and its subsequent depletion of substance P from C fibres takes between 1 and 2 weeks for therapeutic efficacy but up to 6 weeks for maximal effect. As the pain starts to subside it would be expected that the patient's anxiety will also, and related functional symptoms of his IBS should start to recede. Close patient contact is important to track and individualise analgesia and anxiolytic activity. Keeping a pain journal may be clinically useful over the first 6 weeks.

If the neuralgic pain is still persisting after 6 weeks, then a change in prescription may be required. This could include pharmaceutical medicines such as antidepressants, corticosteroids and stronger opioids. If the condition worsens then medical referral is advised for specialist neurological consultation. After the neuralgic pain remits, nutritional and herbal treatment (especially adaptogenic, nervous and immune support) can be continued for a further 3–6 months to reduce the chance of relapse.

Clinical pearls

- Herb–drug–nutrient interactions are of higher likelihood in this patient age group and need to be monitored closely. Potential beneficial interactions for analgesia management are possible and require close communication with the primary medical practitioner or specialist.

- Pain management is imperative to secure patient comfort and improve quality of life. The likelihood that this will be achieved solely by herbal or nutritional therapies is unlikely, so an integrative approach may be required.

- Long-term psychological, nervine tonic and adaptogenic support is encouraged due to the prolonged and complex nature of neuropathic pain.

Expert|CONSULT

Clinical Comprehension Questions & Answers are hosted on **https://expertconsult.inkling.com/store/book/ sarris-clinical-naturopathy-case-files-1**

BIBLIOGRAPHY

Backonja M, Wallace MS, Blonsky ER, et al. NGX-4010, a high-concentration capsaicin patch, for the treatment of postherpetic neuralgia: a randomised, double-blind study. *Lancet Neurol.* 2008;7(12):1106-1112.

Caterina MJ, Schumacher MA, Tominaga M, et al. The capsaicin receptor: a heat-activated ion channel in the pain pathway. *Nature.* 1997;389(6653):816-824.

Sinclair J. Pain management. In: Sarris J, Wardle J, eds. *Clinical Naturopathy: An Evidence-Based Guide to Practice.* 2nd ed. Chatswood: Elsevier; 2014:803-822.

Verma P, Dhaliwal K, Walton N. Review of treatment considerations for post-herpetic neuralgia in the elderly. *UTMJ.* 2011;89(1):33-36.

47 Polypharmacy patients

Justin Sinclair

PRESENTATION

A 69-year-old female presents with **severe persistent asthma**, **chronic pain** from bilateral **osteoarthritis** of the knees and **insomnia**. Recent results from a bone scan and blood tests are also suggestive of early-stage **osteoporosis** and **hypercholesterolaemia**. She is currently medicated on **prednisolone, salbutamol, paracetamol with codeine, diazepam** and **atorvastatin**. She asks for advice on which complementary medicines may improve her health and assist her in safely reducing some of her medications.

Diagnostic considerations

Due to the severe presentation of asthma, close medical supervision and open communication channels between all healthcare providers is highly advisable. Specialist pharmacist consultation may also be required if drug–drug interactions are suspected due to polypharmacy. Treatment of the above case should initially focus on evaluating potential drug–drug interactions and adverse effects, management strategies for the osteoarthritis and insomnia and optimising health and vitality. The insomnia may be due to the chronic pain associated with the osteoarthritis and not an independent disease presentation. Naturopathically, establishing conditions for health, removing obstacles to cure, 'tonifying' weakened systems and symptomatic amelioration are high priorities for current treatment.

Dealing with patients taking medications is one of the most challenging areas of complementary medicine practice, especially where polypharmacy is concerned. A methodical and systematic approach (the INQUIRE method: Investigate all aspects of current medications; Note posology of medications; Qualify and rationalise strengths and limitations; Understand the patient and their case history; Identify potential interactions; Remember to refer or contact other healthcare providers where necessary; Educate the patient) to prescribing complementary medicines to patients taking pharmaceutical medications is considered best practice.

COMMONLY ENCOUNTERED DRUGS WITH NARROW THERAPEUTIC RANGES

- Antiarrhythmics (e.g. quinidine and disopyramide)
- Hypoglycaemics (e.g. insulin)
- Antiepileptics/anticonvulsants (e.g. phenytoin and valproic acid)
- Immunosuppressants (e.g. cyclosporine)
- Mood-altering drugs (e.g. lithium carbonate)
- Anti-HIV drugs (e.g. saquinavir)
- Monoamine oxidase inhibitors
- Antineoplastics (e.g. methotrexate)
- Opioid analgesics
- Barbiturates
- Theophylline
- Cardiac glycosides (e.g. digoxin)
- Tricyclic antidepressants

Treatment protocol

- Baseline blood tests can be ordered to assess age-related changes to organ function including liver and kidney function tests, blood glucose, blood lipids and full blood evaluation. These are important to consider when it comes to drug metabolism and clearance rates.

- A detailed medication review is essential. Assessment for side effects, toxicity, drug–drug interactions and pharmacodynamic/pharmacokinetic/physicochemical mechanisms need to be fully elucidated. This forms the foundation for safe herb and nutrient selection.

- After medical consultation, systemic prednisolone usage can be reduced slowly in a tapered manner. This must be done to reduce the likelihood of sudden severe withdrawal symptoms (e.g. adrenal crisis) and can be replaced with an inhaled corticosteroid (e.g. beclomethasone, budesonide or fluticasone) under the guidance of their prescribing medical practitioner.

- Short-acting β_2-adrenergic receptor agonist reliever medication such as salbutamol (4–6 hour coverage) may be used as required. Salmeterol (long-acting β_2-adrenergic receptor agonist) can be introduced by the medical practitioner daily to provide longer periods (12 hours) of cover.

- During the period of prednisolone withdrawal, the patient should be making weekly contact with their medical practitioner for monitoring.

Compliance and patient education are reinforced as being crucial for positive outcomes.

- In this case, long-term administration of prednisolone was considered a potential contributing factor to the early osteoporosis. Calcium supplementation, along with vitamin D, can be started immediately.

- Long-term reliance on paracetamol with codeine for analgesia increases the potential for habit formation and tolerance. Abruptly stopping this medication may cause a substantial increase in perceived pain. Naproxen sodium (250 mg 4 × daily) or ibuprofen (200 mg 4 × daily) may be introduced to replace paracetamol/codeine initially if required.

- Glucosamine sulfate (GS) may be started for its anti-inflammatory and chondroprotective activity. Pain relief from responders to GS usually occurs within 6 weeks. Naproxen sodium could address pain relief until the GS and herbal prescription take effect, at which time it may be used as rescue medication only.

- *Harpagophytum procumbens, Zingiber officinale* and *Curcuma longa* may be beneficial as herbal anti-inflammatories. The latter two may also confer gastroprotective (anti-ulcer) activity to counter the side effects of nonsteroidal anti-inflammatory drugs.

- Reducing acid-forming foods in the diet is to be encouraged, with increases in alkaline foods such as fresh fruit and vegetables.

- Zostrix (capsaicin 0.025%) topical cream can provide quick relief for joint pain.

- Much akin to systemic corticosteroids, diazepam should not be stopped abruptly due to side effects. The dosage of diazepam can be tapered down by the medical practitioner. A standardised soporific herbal formula (*Valeriana officinalis* equiv. dry root 1.25 g and *Humulus lupulus* equiv. dry fruit 360 mg) can be utilised to address the patient's insomnia during this time. A potential beneficial pharmacodynamic interaction is possible.

- Statin withdrawal can be withheld until the patient is stabilised on their new treatment plan and new blood tests are acquired. The herbal formulation in the initial treatment plan carries secondary advantages because *Zingiber officinale* and *Curcuma longa* are known hypocholesterolaemics, which may require a reduction in statin dosage. Coenzyme Q10 can be administered to address the known depletion caused by HMG-CoA-reductase inhibitors.

PRESCRIPTION
Herbal formula (100 mL)

Harpagophytum procumbens 1:2	50 mL
Curcuma longa 1:1	35 mL
Zingiber officinale 1:2	15 mL

Dose: 5 mL 3 × daily before meals

Standardised *Valeriana officinalis/Humulus lupulus* formulation: 1–2 tablets (before bed)

Zostrix (capsaicin 0.025%) topical analgesic cream (apply 3–4 × daily to affected area)

Nutritional prescription

Glucosamine sulfate: 750 mg 2 × daily

Calcium (hydroxyapatite): 500 mg 3 × daily

Co-Q10 (ubiquinone): 100 mg 2 × daily

Lifestyle prescription

Gentle exercise

Mindfulness meditation

Good sleep hygiene

Dietary improvement

Expected outcomes and follow-up protocols

When patients are 'coming off' pharmaceutical medications, close medical and naturopathic supervision is required. Changes in pain perception, mental status or newly-presenting clinical features must be followed up quickly. In the above case, the patient's asthma would be expected to improve within 2–4 weeks as the long-acting β2-agonists in combination (ICS/LABA) provide more therapeutic coverage. Herbal medicines, with the inclusion of Zostrix, should see improvement in arthritis pain within 4–7 days, with maximum effect from the glucosamine taking up to 6 months. This improvement should warrant more gentle exercise, improving patient quality of life and reducing disease progression. Insomnia, while being removed with diazepam, follows a less predictable clinical trajectory and must be managed closely in a multidisciplinary approach.

Clinical pearls

- It is never appropriate for a non-medical practitioner to advise a patient to stop taking prescribed medications. Any dosage adjustment must be done by the prescribing medical practitioner.

- Patients should be counselled to avoid self-medicating with nutritional and herbal medicines without prior approval.

- Always make the investigation of pharmaceutical medications a priority at the *start* of the consult. This way you can have a clear picture of what signs or symptoms might be drug side effects as opposed to actual diseases or conditions.

Expert | CONSULT

Clinical Comprehension Questions & Answers are hosted on https://expertconsult.inkling.com/store/book/ sarris-clinical-naturopathy-case-files-1

BIBLIOGRAPHY

Coxeter PD, McLachlan AJ, Duke CC, et al. Herb-drug interactions: an evidence-based approach. *Curr Med Chem.* 2004;11:1513-1525.

Sinclair J, Sinclair C. Polypharmacy and drug-nutraceutical interactions. In: Sarris J, Wardle J, eds. *Clinical Naturopathy: An Evidence-Based Guide to Practice.* 2nd ed. Chatswood: Elsevier; 2014:823-838.

Sinclair J. Polypharmacy and pain management. In: Sarris J, Wardle J, eds. *Clinical Naturopathy: An Evidence-Based Guide to Practice.* Chatswood: Elsevier; 2010:736-749.

Stargrove M, Treasure J, McKee D. *Herb, Nutrient and Drug Interactions – Clinical Implications and Therapeutic Strategies.* St Louis: Mosby; 2007.

Index

Page numbers followed by '*b*' indicate boxes.

comorbid ADHD, bipolar disorder with
  (continued)
  follow-up protocols of, 62–63
  prescription for, 62*b*
  treatment protocol of, 61–62
comorbid depression, 40–44
comorbid insomnia, chronic anxiety with, 64–68,
  64*b*
  clinical pearls, 67*b*
  diagnostic considerations of, 64–65, 65*b*
  expected outcomes of, 66–67
  follow-up protocols of, 66–67
  prescription for, 67*b*
  treatment protocol of, 65–66
constipation
  functional, 6–9, 6*b*
    clinical pearls, 9
    diagnostic considerations of, 7
    expected outcomes of, 8–9
    follow-up protocols of, 8–9
    prescription for, 8*b*
    treatment protocol of, 7–8
  in nocturnal enuresis, 207
cortisol level, and hypothalamic-pituitary
  function, 89
Corydalis ambigua
  for dysmenorrhoea, 107, 108*b*
  for general menstrual complaints, 124
  for pain management, 224–225, 225*b*
  for rheumatoid arthritis, 146
counselling, for dysmenorrhoea, 107–108,
  108*b*
cramping, heavy, 118
Crataegus oxyacantha, 51
  cardiovascular disease and, 41–42
  hypertension and, 46–47
Curcuma longa, 16–18, 22, 23*b*, 32, 214
  bowel cancer and, 191
  cardiovascular disease and, 43
  for CFS, 83*b*
  for polypharmacy patients, 229, 230*b*
  for rheumatoid arthritis, 146–147
curcumin, for prostate cancer, 197, 197*b*
cyclic-AMP (cAMP), psoriasis and, 171
Cynara scolymus, 22, 23*b*, 51
  cardiovascular disease and, 41–42

D
deep vein thrombosis (DVT), 54
defecation, in dysmenorrhoea, 107–108, 108*b*
depression
  ageing and, 77
  clinical, CFS and, 82, 82*b*

depression *(continued)*
  comorbid, 40–44
  in elevated HPL concentrations, 219
depurative herbs, for hormonal acne, 176
dermatitis, medical conditions that may mimic,
  171*b*
diarrhoea, 10
  medical conditions associated with or
    aggravate, 11*b*
diarrhoea-predominant irritable bowel syndrome,
  2–5, 2*b*
  clinical pearls, 5
  diagnostic considerations of, 2–3
  expected outcomes of, 4–5
  follow-up protocols of, 4–5
  medical conditions may present as, 3*b*
  prescription for, 4*b*
  treatment protocol of, 3–4
dietary advice
  in assisted reproduction, 132–133
  in erectile dysfunction, 51
  in nocturnal enuresis, 208–209
dietary modifications
  for malvaria, 220
  for metabolic syndrome, 101, 102*b*
dietary triggers, gastro-oesophageal reflux disease
  and, 8
diindolylmethane (DIM), for hormonal acne,
  175
dioxins, and endocrine function, 89
docosahexaenoic acid (DHA), hypertension and,
  46
DVT *see* deep vein thrombosis
dysbiosis, 3
dyslipidaemia, 50
dysmenorrhoea, 106–109, 106*b*
  clinical pearls in, 109
  diagnostic considerations in, 106–107
  expected outcomes in, 108–109
  follow-up protocols in, 108–109
  as general menstrual complaint, 122
  prescription for, 108*b*
  symptoms of, conditions that may mimic, 107*b*
  treatment protocol of, 107–108
dyspnoea, in HIV, 212–213

E
eating habits, modifications of, for metabolic
  syndrome, 101
Echinacea angustifolia, recurrent urinary tract
  infections and, 185
Echinacea purpurea, 213–214
Echinacea root blend, for CFS, 83*b*

glutamine powder, for CFS, 83*b*
glycated haemoglobin (HbA$_{1C}$), for metabolic
    syndrome, 103
glycosides, in polypharmacy patients, 228*b*
Glycyrrhiza glabra, 16, 32, 116, 208
    for CFS, 83*b*
    for endometriosis, 111
    for generalised stress and fatigue, 96–97
goitrogenic foods, for hypothyroidism, 90
GORD *see* gastro-oesophageal reflux disease
GOS *see* galacto-oligosaccharides
guided imagery, in nocturnal enuresis, 209
GUT repair powder formula, 214
Gymnema sylvestre, 22, 23*b see also* chromium

H

Harpagophytum procumbens, 142*b*
    for polypharmacy patients, 229, 230*b*
    for rheumatoid arthritis, 146
headache, 73
    tension and migraine, 155–159, 155*b*
        clinical pearls of, 159
        diagnostic considerations of, 155–156
        expected outcomes of, 158–159
        follow-up protocols of, 158–159
        prescription of, 158*b*
        treatment protocol of, 157
Helicobacter pylori, 76
Hemidesmus indicus, for rheumatoid arthritis,
    146–147
hepatic herbs, for hormonal acne, 175
herbal formula
    for acute upper respiratory tract infection,
        29–30
    for allergies and eczema, 164*b*
    for asthma, 33*b*
    for chronic anxiety, 67*b*
    for chronic sinusitis, 37*b*
    for chronic venous insufficiency, 56*b*
    for clinical depression, 71
    for diarrhoea-predominant irritable bowel
        syndrome, 4*b*
    for erectile dysfunction, 52*b*
    for gastro-oesophageal reflux disease, 8*b*
    for general menstrual complaints, 125
    for generalised stress and fatigue, 97
    for migraine (nervous), 75
    for NAFLD, 23
    for nocturnal enuresis, 209*b*
    for osteoarthritis and myofascial pain
        syndrome, 141–142, 142*b*
    for paediatric immune dysregulation, 204
    for PCOS, 120

herbal formula *(continued)*
    for perimenopausal patients, 129*b*
    for prostate cancer, 197, 197*b*
    for subfertility, 137
herbal infusion, for chronic sinusitis, 37*b*
herbal medicinal tea, recurrent urinary tract
    infections and, 185–186
herbal medicines
    in assisted reproduction, 132–133
    for dysmenorrhoea, 107, 108*b*
    for metabolic syndrome, 102, 102*b*
herbal tablet, for asthma, 33*b*
herbal tea therapies, for NAFLD, 22
herbs
    adaptogenic, for hormonal acne, 176
    depurative, for hormonal acne, 176
    hepatic, for hormonal acne, 175
hereditary factors, in general menstrual
    complaints, 123
high-density lipoprotein, 40
high-intensity interval training (HIIT), for
    metabolic syndrome, 100
hirsutism, reduction of, 120
HIV, 212–216, 212*b*, 215*b*
    clinical pearls, 215
    diagnostic considerations of, 212–213
    expected outcomes and, 214–215
    follow-up protocols for, 214–215
    prescription for, 215*b*
    symptoms of, 213*b*
    treatment protocol of, 213–214
hormonal acne, 174–177
    diagnosis of, other conditions to consider in,
        175*b*
    diagnostic considerations for, 174–175
    expected outcomes and follow-up protocol
        for, 177
    prescription for, 176*b*
    presentation of, 174*b*
    treatment protocol for, 175–176
hormonal factors, in general menstrual
    complaints, 123
hormonal imbalance, disorder of, 110
HPA *see* hypothalamic-pituitary-adrenal (HPA)
    axis
HPO *see* hypothalamic-pituitary-ovarian (HPO)
    axis
Humulus lupus, for sleep and anxiety, 79*b*
Hydrastis canadensis, 27, 29*b*, 30, 34, 74, 75*b*,
    213
hydration
    for acute upper respiratory tract infection, 28
    importance of, 185

omega-3 fatty acids *(continued)*
  polyunsaturated, 51
  for prostate cancer, 198
opioid analgesics, in polypharmacy patients, 228*b*
oral contraceptive pill (OCP), and hormonal
  acne, 174*b*
osteoarthritis, myofascial pain syndrome and,
  140–144, 140*b*
  clinical pearls, 143
  diagnostic considerations of, 140–141
  expected outcomes and, 142–143
  follow-up protocols for, 142–143
  medical conditions of, 141*b*
  prescription for, 142*b*
  treatment protocol for, 141–142
ovarian maturation, thyroid gland and, 88–89
overweight, as factors in PCOS, 118
oxidative stress, metabolic syndrome with, 100

P

paediatric immune dysregulation, 202–206,
  202*b*
  clinical pearls, 206
  diagnostic considerations of, 202–203
  expected outcomes and, 205–206
  follow-up protocols for, 205–206
  naturopathic treatment aims in, 203*b*
  prescription for, 204*b*
  treatment protocol for, 203–205, 205*b*
PAF *see* platelet-activating factor
pain
  common conditions manifesting, 224*b*
  definition of, 223
  diagnostic considerations in, 223–224
  management of, 223–226, 223*b*
    clinical pearls, 226
    prescription for, 225*b*
  reduction
    for dysmenorrhoea, 108, 122
    for endometriosis, 112
    rheumatoid arthritis and, 145
    treatment protocol for, 224–225
Panax ginseng, 129
  for ageing and cognition, 79*b*
  for generalised stress and fatigue, 96–97
  for hypothyroidism, 91
Panax notoginseng, 116
pancreatin digest mucus accumulations, 36
papain, 36
Passiflora incarnata, 65–66, 70, 71*b*, 208
  for sleep and anxiety, 78
patient education, for metabolic syndrome,
  100–102

PCOS *see* polycystic ovarian syndrome
Pelargonium sidoides, 27, 29*b*, 30, 32, 36, 203,
  204*b*
perimenopausal patients, 127–130, 127*b*
  clinical pearls and, 130
  diagnostic considerations of, 127–128
  expected outcomes and, 129–130
  follow-up protocols for, 129–130
  prescription for, 129*b*
  symptoms of, 128*b*
  treatment protocol for, 128–129
periods, irregular, 118
Petasites hybridus, 74
phantom pain, 224*b*
physical activity, for benign prostatic hypertrophy,
  181–182
physical medicine, for osteoarthritis and
  myofascial pain syndrome, 142, 142*b*
physiological pain, 224*b*
phytate-containing vegetables, in fibroids, 115
phyto-oestrogens, 110
Piper methysticum, 3–4, 65–66, 128–129
  chronic anxiety and, 66
  for sleep and anxiety, 78
platelet-activating factor (PAF), 31
PMS *see* premenstrual syndrome
polychlorinated biphenyls, and endocrine
  function, 89
polycystic ovarian syndrome (PCOS), 118–121,
  166–167
  clinical pearls for, 121
  diagnostic considerations in, 118
  expected outcomes of, 119–121
  follow-up protocols for, 119–121
  prescription for, 120*b*
  presentation of, 118*b*
  symptoms of, mimic or aggravate, 119*b*
  treatment protocol for, 119
polypharmacy patients, 227–231, 227*b*
  clinical pearls, 231
  diagnostic considerations in, 227–228,
    228*b*
  expected outcomes in, 230
  follow-up protocols in, 230
  prescription for, 230*b*
  treatment protocol for, 228–229
polyphenols, in ageing and cognition, 78
pomegranate, for prostate cancer, 197*b*
positive social interaction, chronic anxiety and,
  66
powdered *Curcuma longa*, for osteoarthritis and
  myofascial pain syndrome, 142*b*
powdered slippery elm (*Ulmus rubra*) bark, 7–8